ESSENTIALS OF CLINICAL MRI

SERIES IN RADIOLOGY

J. Odo Op den Orth, The Standard Biphasic-Contrast Examination of the Sto-mach and Duodenum: Method, Results and Radiological Atlas.
1979. ISBN 90 247 2159 8

J.L. Sellink and R.E. Miller, Radiology of the Small Bowel. Modern Enterocly-sis Technique and Atlas.
1981. ISBN 90 247 2460 0

R.E. Miller and J. Skucas, The Radiological Examination of the Colon. Practi-cal Diagnosis.
1983. ISBN 90 247 2666 2

S. Forgács, Bones and Joints in Diabetes Melitus.
1982. ISBN 90 247 2395 7

G. Németh and H. Kuttig, Isodose Atlas. For Use in Radiotherapy.
1981. ISBN 90 247 2476 7

J. Chermet, Atlas of Phlebography of the Lower Limbs, including the Iliac Veins.
1982. ISBN 90 247 2525 9

B. Janevski, Angiography of the Upper Extremity.
1982. ISBN 90 247 2684 0

M.A.M. Feldberg, Computed Tomography of the Retroperitoneum. An Ana-tomical and Pathological Atlas with Emphasis on the Fascial Planes.
1983. ISBN 0 89838 573 3

L.E.H. Lampmann, S.A. Duursma and J.H.J. Ruys, CT Densitometry in Osteo-porosis. The Impact on Management of the Patient.
1984. ISBN 0 89838 633 0

J.J. Broerse and T.J. MacVittie, Response of Different Species to Total Body Irradiation.
1984. ISBN 0 89838 678 0

C. L'Herminé, Radiology of Liver Circulation.
1985. ISBN 0 89838 715 9

G. Maatman, High-resolution Computed Tomography of the Paranasal Sinuses, Pharynx and Related Regions.
1986. ISBN 0 89838 802 3

C. Plets, A.L. Baert, G.L. Nijs and G. Wilms, Computer Tomographic Imaging and Anatomic Correlation of the Human Brain.
1986. ISBN 0 89838 811 2

J. Valk, MRI of the Brain, Head, Neck and Spine. A Teaching Atlas of Clinical Applications.
1987. ISBN 0 89838 957 7

J.L. Sellink, X-Ray Differential Diagnosis in Small Bowel Disease. A Practical Approach.
1987. ISBN 0 89838 351 X

T.H.M. Falke, ed., Essentials of Clinical MRI.
1988. ISBN 0 89838 353 6

ESSENTIALS OF CLINICAL MRI

Edited by

THEO H.M. FALKE
Department of Diagnostic Radiology,
University Hospital Leiden, The Netherlands

1988 **MARTINUS NIJHOFF PUBLISHERS**
a member of the KLUWER ACADEMIC PUBLISHERS GROUP
DORDRECHT / BOSTON / LANCASTER

Distributors

for the United States and Canada: Kluwer Academic Publishers, P.O. Box 358, Accord Station, Hingham, MA 02018-0358, USA
for the UK and Ireland: Kluwer Academic Publishers, MTP Press Limited, Falcon House, Queen Square, Lancaster LA1 1RN, UK
for all other countries: Kluwer Academic Publishers Group, Distribution Center, P.O. Box 322, 3300 AH Dordrecht, The Netherlands

Library of Congress Cataloging in Publication Data

Essentials of clinical MRI.

  (Series in radiology)
  1. Magnetic resonance imaging. I. Falke, Theo H. M.,
1951-   . II. Series. [DNLM: 1. Nuclear Magnetic
Resonance--diagnostic use. WN 445 E78]
RC78.7.N83E845 1988   616.07'54   87-28210

ISBN-13: 978-94-010-7972-3   e-ISBN-13: 978-94-009-3279-1
DOI: 10.1007/978-94-009-3279-1

Book information

This publication is based on a Boerhaave course organized by the Faculty of Medicine, University of Leiden, The Netherlands

TABLE OF CONTENTS

VI

Introduction

I am particularly pleased to be able to write the introduction to this book that resulted from a collaborative effort by the Radiology Department, under the auspices of the Boerhaave Committee for Postgraduate Medical Education of the Faculty of Medicine, at the University of Leiden and the Department of Medical Imaging and Radiological Sciences at Vanderbilt University.

Magnetic resonance imaging affords the opportunity to interrogate organ and system structure and function in a nondestructive manner without serious biological implications. Tissue contrast with this modality is exquisite and inherently superior to that of x-ray computed tomography. The advances to improve signal capture, development of rapid data acquisition techniques, fabrication of more appropriate pulse sequences, and availability of contrast agents portend increased versatility and specificity of these studies.

Despite the proliferation of numerous general and specialized texts, the developments in MRI occur at such a pace that data in these references are necessarily dated. The technical horizon of MRI is vast with almost limitless possibilities of signal generation and plan reconstruction. Tissue contrast is so importantly affected by the coupling of signal generation and capture that collective experience of institutions and investigators is extremely important to the initiate and useful even to those individuals with the greatest clinical experience. We all remain very early on the learning curve and the characteristics of the data is sufficiently unique that direct extrapolation from conventional imaging techniques or even x-ray computed tomography are problematic. MRI represents a journey in uncharted imaging waters.

The authors of this book have attempted to consider the most essential elements of magnetic resonance imaging recognizing they could not be encyclopedic. In general, an organ format has been followed after brief consideration of the basic MRI principles. Other imaging modalities are compared for image content and clinical relevance. Finally, some license will be accorded the presenters as they will be allowed to chose avenues for discussion that they believe hold greatest future promise.

A. Everette James, Jr., J.D., M.D.
Professor and Chairman
Department of Medical Imaging and
Radiological Sciences
Vanderbilt Medical Center
Nashville, Tennessee
USA

CONTRIBUTORS

Baleriaux, D.
   Department of Neuroradiology, Erasmus University Hospital, 808 Route de
   Lennik, B-1070 Brussels, Belgium

Bloem, J.L.
   Department of Radiology, University Hospital, Rijnsburgerweg 10, C2-S,
   2333 AA Leiden, The Netherlands

Buruma, O.J.S.
   Department of Neurology, University Hospital, Rijnsburgerweg 10,
   2333 AA Leiden, The Netherlands

Bydder, G.M.
   Department of Diagnostic Radiology, Royal Postgraduate Medical School,
   Hammersmith Hospital, Ducane Road, London W12 OHS, United Kingdom

Doornbos, J.
   Department of Radiology, University Hospital, Rijnsburgerweg 10, C2-S,
   2333 AA Leiden, The Netherlands

Falke, T.H.M.
   Department of Radiology, University Hospital, Rijnsburgerweg 10, C2-S,
   2333 AA Leiden, The Netherlands

Guit, G.L.
   Department of Radiology, University Hospital, Rijnsburgerweg 10, C2-S,
   2333 AA Leiden, The Netherlands

Heindel, W.
   Radiologisches Institut der Universität Köln, Joseph Steltzmann Strasse
   9, 5000 Koln 41, West Germany

Husband, J.
   CRC CT Scanning Unit Royal Marsden Hospital, Downs Road, Sutton, Surrey
   SM2 5PT, United Kingdom

Kessing, P.H.L.
   Department of Radiology, University Hospital, Rijnsburgerweg 10, C2-SS,
   2333 AA Leiden, The Netherlands

Kessler, R.
   Department of Radiology and Radiological Sciences, Vanderbilt
   University Medical Centre, Nashville, TN 37232, U.S.A.

Kieft, G.J.
   Department of Radiology, University Hospital, Rijnsburgerweg 10, C2-S,
   2333 AA Leiden, The Netherlands

Kramer, P.P.G.
   Department of Radiology, University Hospital, Catharijnesingel 101, 3583
   CP Utrecht, The Netherlands

Luiten, A.L.
    Philips Medical Systems Division, P.O. Box 10.000, 5680 DA Best, The
    Netherlands

McNamara, M.T.
    Division of MRI, Princess Grace Hospital, 9800 Principality of Monaco,
    Monaco

Mazer, M.
    Department of Radiology and Radiological Sciences, Vanderbilt
    University Medical Centre, Nashville, TN 37232, U.S.A.

Rohmer, J.
    Department of Pediatric Cardiology, University Hospital, Rijnsburgerweg
    10, 2333 AA Leidenm, The Netherlands

De Roos, A.
    Department of Radiology, University Hospital, Rijnsburgerweg 10, CS-2,
    2333 AA Leiden, The Netherlands

De Slegte, R.G.M.
    Department of Radiology and Neuroradiology, Free University, De
    Boelelaan 1117, 1081 HV Amsterdam, The Netherlands

Taminiau, A.H.M.
    Department of Orthopaedic Surgery, University Hospital, Rijnsburgerweg
    10, 2333 AA Leiden, The Netherlands

Vielvoye, G.J.
    Department of Radiology, University Hospital, Rijnsburgerweg 10, C2-S,
    2333 AA Leiden, The Netherlands

Voormolen, J.H.C.
    Department of Neurosurgery, University Hospital, Rijnsburgerweg 10, 2333
    AA Leiden, The Netherlands

Van Voorthuisen, A.E.
    Department of Radiology, University Hospital, Rijnsburgerweg 10, C2-S,
    2333 AA Leiden, The Netherlands

Ziedses des Plantes Jr., B.G.
    Department of Radiology, St. Geertruiden Hospital, H.J.P. Fesevurstraat
    7, 7415 CM Deventer, The Netherlands

ACKNOWLEDGMENT

This study was partly supported by the Dutch Cancer Foundation, Grant IKW 85-89.
We thank Schering AG Berlin (FRG), in particular Dr. W. Clauss for supplying gadolinium (Gd-DTPA) meglumine.

Particular appreciation is due to my secretary, Fokje Noorderijk for wide ranging support with the manuscript preparation and secretarial assistance.
Gerrit Kracht has our thanks for the photography.

Most of all I am grateful to my fellow radiologists whose interest and continuing support in my work has led to the production of this book.

SECTION I GENERAL PRINCIPLES

SECTION 1. GENERAL NOTES

BASIC FACTS AND RECENT DEVELOPMENTS IN MR IMAGING

A.L. LUITEN

1. INTRODUCTION

Some 15 years ago the physical principle of NMR spectroscopy, which again was discovered some 25 years earlier, was applied for the first time to obtain a cross-sectional image of water containing objects, in particular of biological tissues. It showed the intensity distribution of the emitted proton resonance radiation. This was the birth of the proton spin imaging or the magnetic resonance imaging.

During the last ten years a rapid development of the technical possibilities and the medical application has taken place with an ever increasing rate. Continuously new imaging procedures are being published. The flexibility and the quality of imaging techniques has improved enormously. Flow and motion phenomena can be studied now by angiographic methods and movie techniques. The last technique is stimulated strongly by the introduction of faster imaging methods that have recently extended the field MRI applications with new possibilities, such as dynamic studies of the heart and renal function.

Finally the new possibilities created by a combination of imaging techniques and NMR spectroscopy may lead in the near future to a new diagnostic tool: in-vivo spatially localized spectroscopy (MRS), of which the first application studies are presently being carried out.

2. PRINCIPLES OF MRI

An externally applied magnetic field (Bo) exerts an aligning influence on those atomic nuclei that possess a magnetic moment. This effect is called the nuclear magnetization of the material (FIG. Ib).

In human tissues this primarily concerns, the nuclei of hydrogen (1H), sodium (23N) and phosphor (31P).

The existence of an aligned equilibrum orientation of these nuclei also introduces the possibility of vibration and resonance, somewhat analogous to the properties of the strings of an musical instrument. Application during a short period of time of a hf magnetic field of the right frequency and perpendicular to the static field Bo and brings the nuclei in an excited state. They re-emit the absorbed energy as resonance radiation (FIG. 1c and d).

Super imposing on Bo a static weak inhomogeneous magnetic field produced by a set of auxiliary coils (gradient coils) can make that the frequency and the phase of the resonance radiation are labeled by the spatial coordinates of the emitting nucleus.

Out of a number (e.g. 256) of received resonance signals with different spatial encoding of frequency or phase the spectrometer can extract the spatial information needed to perform the computer reconstruction of the 2- or 3- dimensional image of the object cross-section or total volume. A principle MR imaging is possible with all nuclei with a magnetic moment.

However, because of the high concentration and relatively high signal strengths of protons in comparison to other relevant nuclei (Na, P). MRI is practically exclusively applied on the hydrogen nuclei of the water and fat molecules in the human body.

3. CHARACTERISTIC PROPERTIES OF MRI TECHNIQUES
3.1 Emission tomography
The radiation originates from the hydrogen nuclei present in the object and can only be increased by a higher fieldstrength B_0, which increases the degree of nuclear alignment or the nuclear magnetization.

Images of higher resolution have less protons per pixel and are consequently more noisy. The noise can be suppressed by averaging of the signals of repeated measurements but this leads to a corresponding increase in measuring time.

3.2 Limited repetition rate of measurements
During each measurement magnetization is partly or fully destroyed and a certain magnetic recovery time is needed between the successive measurements. A repetition time TR shorter than the magnetization time constant T1, which is strongly tissue dependent (0.1 - 1.5 sec.), yields weaker resonance signals and thus more noisy images.

Routinely used repetition times of 0.5 to 1 sec. leads to image recording times of 5 to 15 minutes.

3.3 Free selectable orientation of the images cross-section (FIG. 2)
A static gradient field applied during the RF excitation pulse makes the B_0 field inhomogeneous in the gradient direction and results in the selective excitation of only a certain slice of the object perpendicular to the gradient direction.

An appropiate combination of x-, y- and z-gradient enables the imaging of orthogonal planes (transverse coronal, sagittal) as well as any oblique orientation. Different parallel planes can be imaged by only changing the RF excitation frequency. Slice thickness is governed by excitation bandwidth and gradient strength. In principle no patient repositioning is necessary.

3.4 Multiple slice imaging (FIG. 3)
The recovery time between two successive measurements of one slice can be used to perform the similar measurement on a series of other non-intersecting, most often parallel slices with freely selectable interslice spacing. Depending on measuring conditions 2 to 20 or more slices can be imaged in the same time of one single slice.

3.5 Multiple echo imaging (FIG. 4)
Due to the coordinate encoding of the frequency of the resonating protons the received resonance signal is much shorter than the characteristic decay time T2 of the signals emitted by the protons within one pixel.

The gradient field applied during detection of signals cause rapidly increasing phase differencens between different pixels and a corresponding decrease in total signal amplitude.

The signal can however be recalled in the spin-echo technique by either inverting the phase differences through a inverting RF pulse (180°- pulse) or by inverting the gradient direction: respectively the "RF-echo" and the "gradient field echo". This can be repeated a number of times with an exponentially decreasing echo signal strength (T2 relaxation time).

4. CONTRAST EFFECTS

The contrast between various tissues arises from a difference in resonance signal intensity due to different causes:
a. The proton density of different tissues depends on the water concentration which varies from 70 to 100%.
b. The relaxation time T1 creates a magnetization difference determined by
the selected repetition time TR (FIG. 5).
c. the relaxation T2 creates differences in signal intensity decay depending on the selected echo time TE (FIG. 4).
d. Moving protons in a fluid flow may increase the resonance signal if
they possess maximum magnetization when entering into the imaged slice
between two measurements. Motion may also decrease the pixel brightness
if the protons move out of the slice before the end of the echotime TE,
or if dephasing effects occur due to turbulent motion.
e. Chemical shift effect: protons in water have a slightly different resonance frequency (approx. 3 ppm) than protons in fatty acids due to
different chemical environment. This can lead to phase differences
between water and fat signals that can be used to create contrasts depending on the fat-water ratio of the tissue (chemical shift imaging).

Particularly interesting is the recently intorduced application of
contrast media, such as Gadolinium chelate (Gd-DTPA), that strongly shorten the T1 relaxation of the water protons.
Being transported by the blood flow the contrast medium can be used to
depict blood supply, perfusion and transport mechanisms in various organs
(brain, kidney, liver, etc.). It also can create a discrimination between
tumor and edemous tissue, and assist in the diagnoses of infarcts, ischemia, cysts etc.

5. Flow and motion effects

Moving speed of cardiac walls and flow rates of blood can be calculated
by exactly recording the motion induced phase differences between the
signals from stationary and moving protons in the imaged plane. The quantitative flow imaging yields information on flow rates and flow velocity
profiles in the larger blood vessels (aorta).
The qualitative flow imaging yields an angiographic technique. This
mostly includes a subtraction technique of identical images with different
flow dephasing effects. This results in an image only showing the flowing
fluids with suppression of all stationary image details. In the case of
blood one then only sees the blood vessels in a similar fashion as in
X-ray angiography.

6. Fast MR imaging techniques

Normal RF excitation pulses rotate the proton magnetization 90 out of
the aligned orientation. Applying a smaller RF pulse results in flipping
the magnetization over a smaller angle $\propto$. This reduces the signal strength
by a factor $\sin \propto$, but as it conserves a magnetization component of $\cos \propto$,
the magnetization recovery will require less time.
Simultaneous reduction of the repetition time TR now leads to considerable shortening of the measuring time albeit with a reduced but still
practicable signal strength.
Furthermore, the echo time TE is reduced to a minimum in order to minimize the signal decay related to T2 relaxation. The short TE is achieved
by applying gradient reversal echoes instead of more time requiring RF

inversion pulses.

By also decreasing the resolution to 128 pixels one can even obtain scan times of about 3 seconds. The reduced image quality however still appears to be sufficient for a number of purposes, such as an orientation image, a single frame in a movie series, kidney function studies with contrast agents, etc.

The variation of the flip angle α further also strongly influences the image contrast: T2-weighting with small flip angle (20°) and T1-weighting at larger angles (60-90°).

The reduced repetition time also creates the possibility of simultaneous imaging of the heart in a large number of (16 or more) different phases of the heart cycle (fast multiphase imaging). To produce an image 128 or 256 measurements are required and thus the same number of heart cycles recording time is needed.

Contrast media shorten the magnetic recovery time and are therefore very important when using fast imaging techniques. Contrast agents then cause a very bright image contrast and yield the possibility of time function studies of organs such as kidneys.

Three-dimensional imaging with isotropic resolution requires thousands of measurements and thus has now become practicable in combination with fast imaging, which reduces the measuring time by more than a factor of 10 to about 5 or 10 minutes.

7. Spectroscopy

High-resolution NMR spectroscopy is usually applied as a non-destructive analysis of biochemical compounds. In-vivo spectroscopy means the measurement of the chemical composition of a volume element inside the human body. This requires the selection and spatially limitation of the volume of interest which can be achieved by various technical principles derived from the MR imaging techniques.

The spatial localization can be realized by techniques of selective excitation making use of combinations of RF pulses and gradient fields (Bo-techniques), or by combining suitable time series of RF-pulses with a RF surface coil that creates a certain spatially inhomogenous RF field (B1-techniques).

Resonance spectra of 31P and 1H of the metabolites (ADP, PC r, N-Ae, Asp., lactate) are very useful to study the metabolic condition in the cells of the diseased tissue and its response to certain applied stresses or to therapeutic treatments.

Also the study of water and lipid components of the tissue and the analysis of the lipid metabolism are of current interest.

MRS, the medical in-vivo spectroscopy, is still in its early phase of application but may have very important future together with MRI.

7

FIGURE 1. Magnetic resonance of atomic nuclei: a) Random. b) Magnetisation. c) Excitation. d) Relaxation.

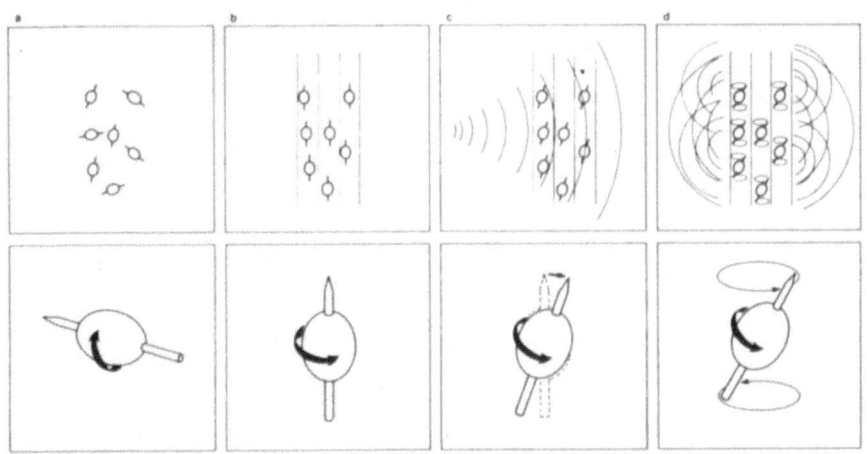

FIGURE 2. Selective excitation of a transverse slice.

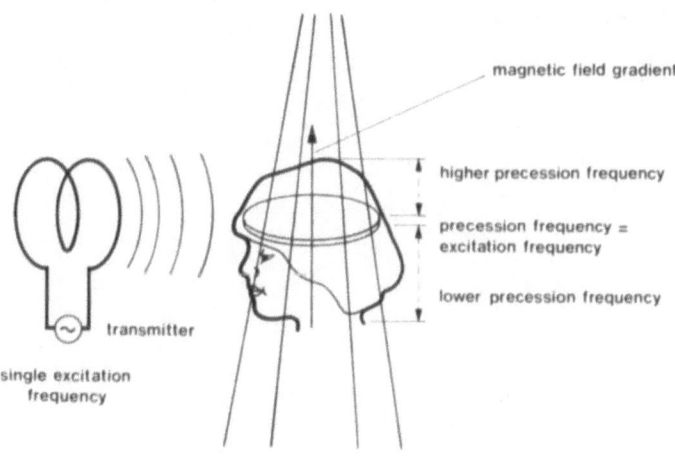

8

FIGURE 3. Simultaneous imaging of a number of slices.

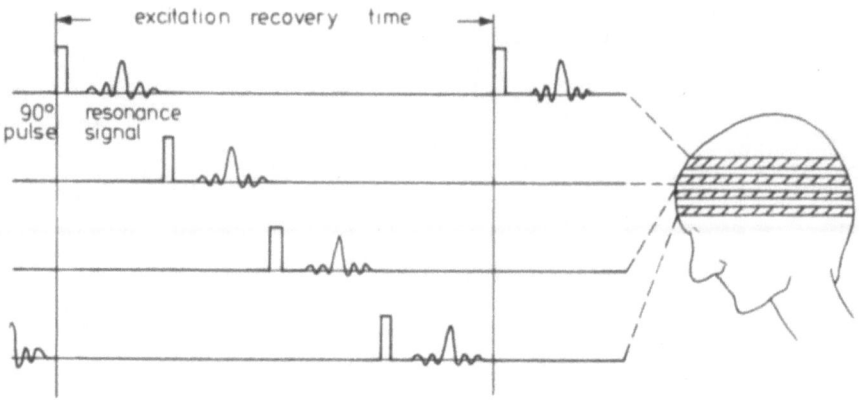

FIGURE 4. Formation of an echo signal with tissue contrast related to signal decay (T2-contrast).

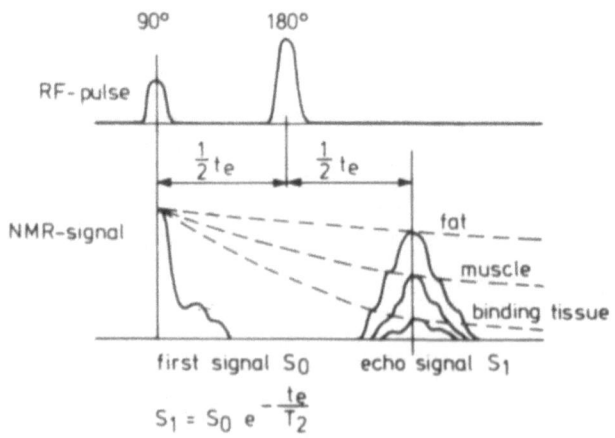

FIGURE 5. Tissue contrast related to incomplete magnetisation (T1-contrast).

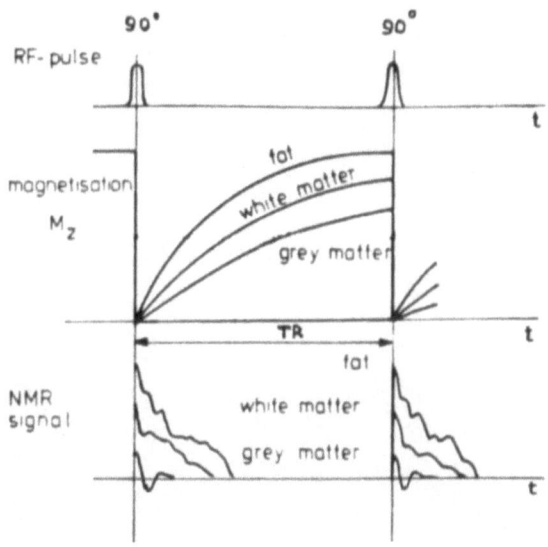

CONTRAST MECHANISMS AND BASIC IMAGE INTERPRETATION
IN MAGNETIC RESONANCE IMAGING

J. DOORNBOS

In magnetic resonance imaging (MRI) tissue contrast is a very important
factor for the diagnostic interpretation of the image. As in other imaging
methods, the appearance of the organs and structures in the body is dependent upon intrinsic tissue properties and extrinsic technical factors [1]. As opposed to many X-ray methods however, MRI can be applied in
various ways, each giving rise to a specific relative tissue brightness in
the image.
Three main tissue properties governing contrast in MRI may be distinguished. First, the so-called spin-lattice and spin-spin MR-relaxation,
characterized by the T1 and T2 time value, respectively. The tissue T1 and
T2 relaxation times reflect the rate of return of the proton spins to
their equilibrium state, after the excitation by a radiofrequency (RF)
pulse. The second important factor is the relative number of hydrogen
nuclei (protons) present in the tissue: the proton density. Furthermore
image contrast is influenced by motion, e.g. flow of blood or cerebrospi-
nal fluid, and diffusion.
Each tissue type has more or less specific T1 and T2 values. However, the
large spread of relaxation times measured in a specific tissue within a
group of patients, and the overlap of these values in normal and diseased
tissue, has hitherto impeded useful tissue characterization based on T1
and T2 values.
Apart from the influence of intrinsic tissue features, image contrast is
a result of the technical factors concerning the examination method which
may be determined by the examinator. In this paper we only consider the
'spin echo' (SE) examination technique and its contrast generating properties. The spin echo technique is the most common pulse sequence applied
in MRI today. The method consists of a series of RF pulses which is repeated a large number of times in order to acquire sufficient information.
The sequence is made up of two pulses, namely the observation-pulse and
the echo-pulse. The time delay between the observation-pulse and the observation is called the 'echo-time' (TE). TE lies usually in the range of
20 - 200 ms. The time between two consecutive pulse sequences is labelled
'repetition-time' (TR) and it usually ranges from 250 ms to 2500 ms.
The intensity (Int) of a picture element in an image obtained via the SE
method is mathematically described by the following approximative equation:

$$Int = N(H).[1-exp(-TR/T1)].exp(-TE/T2) \qquad (Eq. 1)$$

where $N(H)$ is the local proton density.
Intensity changes caused by flow or tissue motion are not accounted for by
this equation. Since most soft tissues contain 80-90% water, i.e. the
proton densities are only slightly differing, the ratios TR/T1 and TE/T2
are the contrast dominating factors in these tissues. For sake of simplicity, we therefore reduce Eq. 1 to

$$Int = A \times B \qquad (Eq. 2)$$
where $A = [1-exp(-TR/T1)]$ and $B = exp(-TE/T2)$.

In the daily practice of MRI most patient examinations are performed by the application of two different pulse sequences. First, an SE sequence with a short TR and TE value is applied: roughly spoken the factor B in Eq. 2 will now equal one, and the observed intensities are predominantly a function of the tissue T1 values. Second, an SE pulse sequence with a relatively long TR and TE is used; now the value of the factor A in Eq. 2 approaches unity and the image intensity is merely dependent on the T2 values. The two image types thus obtained are usually identified as T1-weighted and T2-weighted, respectively.

Application of intermediate TR and TE values will give rise to images in which signal intensity is determined by both T1 and T2 differences between the tissues. Images obtained with a very long TR and a very short TE exhibit minimal influence of T1- and T2-relaxation on the image appearance and are hence called 'proton density' images. In the latter images the proton density is the principal contrast determining factor.

Table 1

Relative intensities of some tissues in the brain

T1-weighted	T2-weighted
High signal intensity	
Hemorrhage	Hemorrhage
Fat	Cystic fluid
	CSF
Bone marrow	Edema
	Tumor
	Fat
	Bone marrow
	Gray matter
Edema	White matter
Gray matter	
Tumor	
CSF / cysts	Cortical bone
Cortical bone	Air
Air	
Low signal intensity	

In the following section we will shed some light on the quantitative meaning of the terms 'T1-weighted' and 'T2-weighted'.
Figs 1 and 2 display 'iso-intensity' contours in the T1-T2 plane, calculated via Eq. 2 (the fraction of the maximally obtainable MR-signal is given). T1-T2-pairs that result in equal signal intensity are connected; the resulting isointensity curves have been drawn at regular intervals. In Fig. 1 the intensities which would result for any combination of T1 and T2 by application of an SE sequence with a TR of 250 ms and a TE of 20 ms (SE-250/20) are displayed. Analogously, Fig. 2 shows the iso-intensity curves as a function of T1 and T2 obtained by application of the SE-2500/100 sequence.

```
-----------------------------------------------------
Table 2
-----------------------------------------------------
Relative intensities of some tissues in the body
-----------------------------------------------------
    T1-weighted                 T2-weighted
              High signal intensity
Old blood                   Old blood
Fat                         Water / cysts
Bone marrow                 Tumor
                            Fresh blood
                            Fat
Solid organs                Bone marrow
Tumor
Muscle
Fresh blood                 Solid organs
Water / cysts               Muscle
Fibrous tissue              Fibrous tissue
Cortical bone               Cortical bone
Air                         Air
              Low signal intensity
-----------------------------------------------------
```

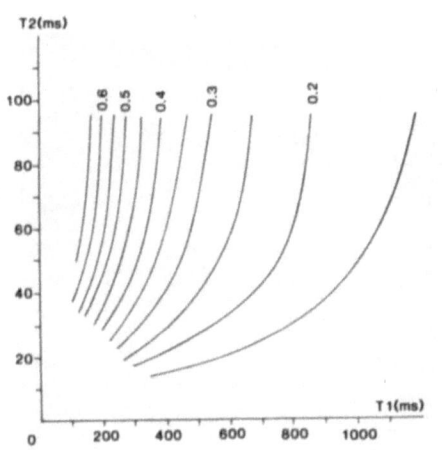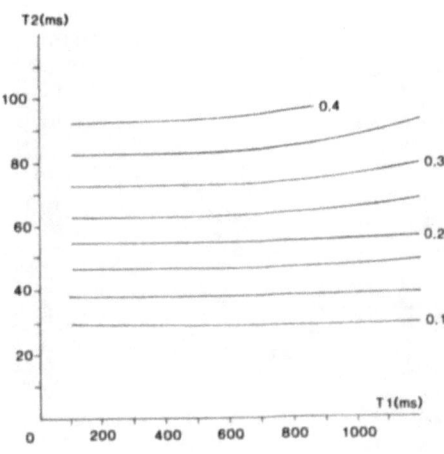

Figure 1   **Figure 2**
Iso-intensity curves plotted in the T1-T2 plane.
Fig.1 T1-weighted pulse sequence SE-250/20
Fig.2 T2-weighted pulse sequence SE-2500/100

The meaning of the terms 'T1-weighted' and 'T2-weighted' may be appreciated from Figs. 1 and 2 in a straightforward manner: 'T1-weighted' means that tissue contrast is primarily dependent on T1 differences between tissues, i.e. T2 differences have little effect on tissue contrast. This is the case in Fig. 1 where the iso-intensity curves are parallel to the T2-axis (except the region of the very short T2 values): a change in T1 will result in a change in intensity, whereas a change in T2 will not. Fig. 2 displays the iso-intensity curves accompanying a T2-weighted pulse sequence. In this case the image intensities change only when T2 varies.

What 'T1-weighted' and 'T2-weighted' means in practice, is visualized in Figs. 3 and 4, these figures give an impression of a transaxial slice of the brain obtained by a T1- and a T2-weighted sequence, respectively.

So far we have not commented upon actual tissue T1 and T2 values in vivo. As stated above, the exact values of the relaxation times exhibit a too large standard deviation to be of general use. However, it is quite possible to categorize tissues into general groups characterized by e.g. a long T1 and T2, a long T1 and short T2, intermediate T1 and T2, etc. So doing, and taking into account the proton density of the tissue (which is important when largely differing body components such as for example lung, bone, liver and urine are imaged), one may construct a table which links tissue types to their intensities in T1- and T2-weighted images- [2-4].

Examples of these schemes are displayed in Table 1 and 2. This type of tables can be set up for any part of the body, and is very informative for the understanding of relative tissue intensities and observed intensity changes caused by e.g. tumor, inflammation, edema or necrosis.

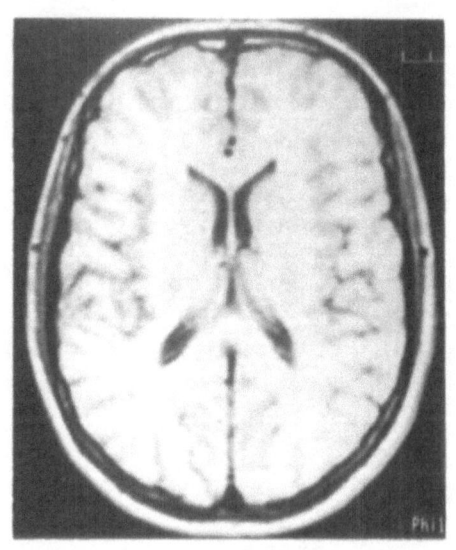 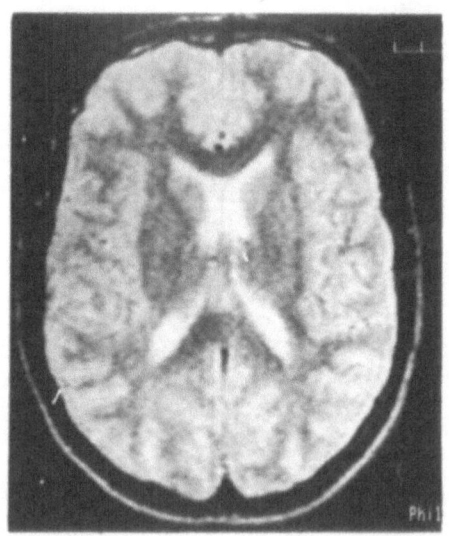

Figure 3   **Figure 4**
MR image of a transaxial slice of the human brain.
Fig. 3 T1-weighted image
Fig. 4 T2-weighted image

However, one should keep in mind that subtle differences in tissue brightness may disappear or even invert when different T1- or T2-weighted techniques are employed. For instance, the SE-250/20 and the SE-600/30 are both called T1-weighted, but these will yield somewhat different tissue contrast.

Notwithstanding this last caveat, summaries of MRI experience as shown in the tables are of great use in basic image interpretation.

REFERENCES
1. B.G. Ziedses des Plantes Jr., T.H.M. Falke, J.A. den Boer. Pulse sequences and contrast in magnetic resonance imaging. Radiographics 4, 869-883 (1984).
2. W.A. Murphy, W.G. Totty. Musculoskeletal Magnetic Resonance Imaging. In "Magnetic Resonance Annual 1986", pp1-36, H.Y. Kressel, ed., Raven Press, New York.
3. M.T. Modic, T.J. Masaryk, and M.A. Weinstein. Magnetic Resonance Imaging of the Spine. In "Magnetic Resonance Annual 1986", pp37-54, H.Y. Kressel, ed., Raven Press, New York.
4. J. Valk et al. 'Basic principles of nuclear magnetic resonance imaging'. Elsevier (1985).

POTENTIAL HAZARDS OF MAGNETIC RESONANCE IMAGING
B.G. ZIEDSES DES PLANTES JR

INTRODUCTION

The greatest hazard associated with Nuclear Magnetic Resonance Imaging (MRI) might be the risk that an incorrect interpretation of the data will result in the wrong therapy being initiated or treatable lesions being ignored (1).
However, in this paper the potential dangers of MRI due to physical effects on the biological system of human beings will be discussed.
The hazards of MR imaging can be divided in three categories:
- The effects of the static magnetic field.
- The effect of electric current induced by the time varying main field.
- The effect of heating by the RF-signal.

STATIC MAGNETIC FIELD

There are 7 effects due to the static field:
- Metal projectiles attracted by the main field.
- Traction on ferromagnetic prothesis.
- Cardiac pace-makers.
- Changes in enzymee kinetics by confirmational changes.
- Magneto haemodynamic interactions.
- Induced electrical currents and voltages in the cardiovascular system.

- Metal projectiles attracted by the main field.
Ferromagnetic objects are attracted by the magnetic field. The force is proportional to the field strength, to the field gradient and to the mass of the object. Very little imagination is needed to consider the effect of a projectile flying into the magnet. The danger of these projectiles is increaséd by the fact that the ferromagnetic objects aligne themselves along the axis of the magnetic field. As a result sharp instruments like a pair of scissors will travel in a longitudinal position with its point directed forwards or backwards.

To our knowledge no serious injuries have been reported in literature. However, most people working with MR imaging are aware of near accidents with flying projectiles. The rules of entering the scanning room must be very stringent. Not only wheel-chairs, stretchers and (small) ferromagnetic instruments must be kept out of the scanning room, but even at night untrained cleaning personnel (with iron buckets) must be prevented from entering the room.
In case of a cardiovascular calamity the patient should be removed as quickly as possible outside the scanning room and resuscitation should take place outside the 5 mTesla line (2).

- Traction on ferromagnetic implants.
Force exerted on ferromagnetic implants can create a danger for the patient. The longitudinal force is proportional to the spatial gradient of the magnetic field and to the magnetization component lying parallel to

the direction of the gradient. The torque is proportional to the field strength itself and to the magnetization components orthogonal to the direction of the field.

New et al. demonstrated in 16 out of 21 vascular clips, which were thought to be non-ferromagnetic, a substantial torque and longitudinal force in circumstances comparable to MRI scanning conditions (3).

The same authors described an experiment with 2 aneurysm clips placed on femoral arteries of a rat. Placed at the portal of a 1.44 Tesla magnet one of the two clips was twisted off the artery. Placed near a 0.147 Tesla magnet both clips were rotated markedly, but neither was detached from the artery (3).

The level of risk is not only proportional to the force applied on the implant (the mass, geometry an degree of ferromagnetism of the implant, the fieldstrength and fieldgradient) but also to the anatomical location, the degree of fixation and to the sensitivity of the structures against which the clip is forced.

Prior to MR imaging patients with metallic implants should be screened with a suitable detector. If the implant has proven to be nonmagnetic, even patients who underwent recent implantation of aneurysm clips, can be imaged without risk of injury (4).

- Cardiac pace-makers.
Field strength of greater than 17 mTesla may switch a demand pace-maker to an asynchronous mode. Although the switching effect is not a threat for most patients, it is a potential danger for pace-maker patients.
According to the "labelling guideline" of the U.S. Bureau of Radiologic Health (5) public areas with fields of 0.5 mTesla or greater must be posted with warnings or be access controlled. (The earth magnetic field is 0.06 mTesla). However, Budinger has measured field strength of 0.7 m Tesla in two subway systems (the Bay Area Rapid Transit in San Francisco and METRO in Washington D.C.). The receiver of an ordinary telephone produces 3.5 mTesla. An audio headset can produce 10 mTesla at the surface of the earpiece (6).

These measurements suggest that a guideline of 1 mTesla as a maximum field strength in public areas might be more reasonable than 0.5 mTesla.

Pavlicek found no effect on pace-makers at a field strength below 10m Tesla (7). He advises an upper limit of 10 mTesla.

- Changes in enzyme kinetics by conformational changes.
In some organic molecules superconductivity is present. This superconductivity might be involved in enzyme reaction kinetics. As magnetic fields can revert a superconductor to a normal state, it has been proposed that enzyme reaction rates may be affected by magnetism (8). Although some reduction in reaction kinetics have been reported at fields of 2 Tesla, this effect could not be reproduced in other experiments at 5 to 20 Tesla (9), even though the circumstances of earlier experiments were carefully reproduced. Also other experiments performed with field strength up to 45 Tesla did not show any important effect on enzyme systems (10,11).

- Orientation effects on molecules and some organized cellular structures.
The magnetization energy or interaction energy of a magnetic field is proportional to the square of the field strength.

Molecules and some organized cellular structures have direction varying magnetic susceptibilities (e.g. sickled cells, DNA, retinal rods and liquid crystals). This spacial difference in susceptibility can produce a

turning torque (8).
   The torque is proportional to:
              - the difference in susceptibilities.
              - the orientation of the molecule relative to the field.
              - the field strength squared.
              - the number of coupled units.
With a sufficiently large asymmetry of each unit and a sufficient number
of units, large turning torques can be expected at a field strength even
below 2 Tesla, as was described in experiments on the orientation effects
of retinal rods at 1 Tesla and the alignment of sickle cells at 0.35 Tesla
(12,13). Even the observations on orientation of bacteria and some animals
might be explained by the physical torque (14).

- Effects on nerve conduction velocity.
   A magnetic field effects a moving charge in that field:

$$F=q(V * B)$$

Where F = force; q= charge; V = velocity and B = magnetic field.
In a similar way a magnetic field can influence the moving ions in nerve
tracks, thus the conduction velocity.
Nerve conductive velocity is very sensitive to temperature. The reported
effects on conduction velocity at 1 Tesla can be explained by temperature
effect. At 2 Tesla no influence conduction velocity was found (15).
Liboff calculated with experiments on a squid axon model that 100 Tesla
are needed for a significant current distortion (16).

- Magnetohaemodynamic interactions.
   A stationary magnetic field has an obstructive effect on moving
electrically conductive fluids: electrical voltages and currents are induced by the motion of the fluid in the magnetic field. The magnetic field
interacts with these currents and produces a a force opposite to the fluid
flow. This can result in an increased blood pressure. The retardation effect is proportional to the field strength squared and to the vessel diameter squared. From calculations it is expected that without physiological
compensation of the peripheral vascular resistance a 10 percent change in
blood pressure would occur at 6 Tesla (6). Under normal conditions this
change can be easily compensated by changes in peripheral resistance.

- Induced electrical currents and voltages in the cardiovascular system.
   The induced voltage for a field perpendicular to the flow is proportional to the flow, the field strength and to the vascular diameter.
This induced voltage can be 0.5 mVolt in the aorta.
The effect of these flow induced voltages in the heart and in the large
vessels is dependent on the position in respect to the magnetic field.
The induced potentials in the heart occur in the systole and can be observed as changes in the T-wave of the ECG. These T-wave changes can be
seen at field strengths below 0.3 Tesla (8).

                    RAPIDLY CHANGING MAGNETIC FIELDS. ·

   According to Faradays Law of induction a time varying magnetic field
(rapidly changing gradient fields) generates an electric current.
There are five types of known effects on a human subject (6):

- Stimulation of visual flash sensation
- Stimulation of nerves
- Induction of heart fibrillation
- Electro-shock anaesthesia
- Bone healing

- Stimulation of visual flash sensation.
The electric currents inducted by a rapidly changing magnetic field can induce visual flash sensation (17). These sensations are called magnetic phosphenes.
The induction of phosphenes is not only dependent on the magnetization changing rate, but also on the duration of the stimulus.
Barlow et al found a threshold of $17\mu A/cm$ at 10-30Hz.
The threshold field change for phosphenes induction is 2 - 5 Tesla/sec. However a minimum amplitude of 10 mTesla is needed at a frequency of 20 - 30 Hz. (19).
At a field change of 5 Tesla/sec the duration of a current density must be at least 2 msec. The duration at MRI is 0.2 msec or less.
Field changes of 210 Tesla/sec with a pulse duration of 3 microseconds did not produce phosphene (8).
During a quench of a 1.76 Tesla magnet a decline of 0.13 Tesla/sec was measured by Bore (20). This decline is well below the advised upper limits mentioned above.
The advice of the Bureau of Radiological Health (U.S.FR.D.A) suggesting a maximum field change rate of 3 Tesla/sec is confusing, because the duration time is not concerned (5).
The British Bureau for Radiation Protection advises a maximum rate of field changing at any part of the body of 20 Tesla/sec. for pulses of 10 msec. or longer (21).

- Stimulation of nerves, induction of seizures and of heart fibrillation.
Current densities in mammalian nerve action potential are about 3 mA/cm^2. Currents applied to the head during 300 msec with current densities of 3 mA/cm^2 can produce seizures (8).
The current densities involved in heart fibrillation are 0.1 to 1 mA/cm^2 (22). These current densities are 10000 greater than those produced during normal MRI strategies (8). However, the biological effect is dependent on the waveform, the amplitude, the time duration and the repetition rate (19). Experiments showed no alteration of action potentials by a pulsed magnetic field of 600000 Tesla/sec for 20 microsec and 900 Tesla/sec for 1.5 msec. (28). Below a stimulus threshold value in the range of 3 Tesla/sec no excitation of a nerve-muscle preparation will occur no matter what the pulse duration might be.

The current density is dependent on the loop diameter. A field change of 10 Tesla/sec will produce a current density of 0.55 mA/cm^2 at the periphery of a stainless steel object of a diameter of 10 cm (8).
Buddinger advises a maximum amplitude of the oscillating magnetic field of 5 mTesla at frequencies below 1-200Hz (8).

- Bone healing.
Stimulation of bone healing by induced electric fields using a coil near the fracture site is an accepted method of therapy (24).
Positive bone healing effects are reported when asymmetric pulses with a rise time of 1 microsecond, a current density of 10 microAmpere and a re-

petition rate of 30-60/sec are applied repeatedly during days or weeks. Sinusoidal waveforms as used in MRI have little or no effect in the range of 30-65 Hz (8).

RADIOFREQUENCY EFFECTS

The rapidly oscillating magnetic field of the RF produces current densities. These currents produce heat in the resistive body.
Most of the heating will occur at the surface of the body. The skin will receive the maximum power. The maximum temperature elevation is expected in the subcutaneous tissues.
Hot spots can occur because of variations in dielectric constants at tissue interfaces and of geometry.
However not all the RF power is absorbed by the body. A part of the signal is reflected at the air/tissue interface. This reflectivity might be as high as 60% at the MRI frequencies used.
Another part is transmitted throught the body without any interference with the body. The RF absorption increases with the RF frequency. The penetration depth for biological tissues, the depth at which the power is reduced by $(1/e)^2$, is shown as a function of frequency in Table 1 (8).

Table 1.

Frequency (MHz)	Penetration depth(cm)
1	91
10	22
41	11
100	7

By radiation and evaporation the human body can lose 500 kcal/hr.
For a specific absorbed power of 4 W/kg for 10 minutes, the expected temperature rise is 0.7 C.
The basal metabolic rate for humans is 1.5 W/kg during sleep and the metabolic rate during heavy exercise is 15 W/kg. Therefore a prudent threshold value for MRI studies is 1.5 W/kg for long duration and 4 W/kg for studies of 10 minutes or less. (8).
Recent experiments and calculations performed by E.R. Adair and L.G. Berglund (25) revealed that 8 W/kg is well tolerated by a 70 kg weighted man, wearing only light pyjamas, whose metabolic rate is at the basal level during the MRI procedure. A core temperature rise of less than 1 C was found after an exposure length of 20 minutes. However this was accompanied by a considerable rise in skin blood flow.
The authors advice to preserve an upper limit of 5 W/kg in elderly patients or patients with compromised cardiovascualr response or people under medication regimes whose pharmacological action may interfere with normal thermoregulatory processes.
Absorption by large metallic implants may result in a significant local heating if the blood circulation is limited (26).
However, during normal MR imaging procedures no side effects have been noticed in patients with prosthesis (27,28) and no significant temperature rise in prosthetic heart valves have been measured (29).

CHRONIC EFFECTS

Little is known about the chronic effects of MR imaging (1).
Epidemiologic reports are controversial.
Biologic effects have been reported, but it is questionable if these effects are really caused by the magnetic field or by the RF signal (8).

CONCLUSION

The most important physiological hazards in MRI are the effects of the static field in iatrogenic circumstances:
- The direct mechanical effect of ferromagnetic objects flying into the magnet and injuring the patient.
- The effect on ferromagnetic implants (especially vascular clips)
- The effect on pace-makers.

The other effects do not seem to present a hazard to the patient provided that the field strength, the magnetic field change rate and the RF power applied are below the advised limits. Experiments described in literature demonstrated that the advised limits have safe and broad margins. A vast surpass of these limits is needed before harmful side-effects are noticed.

With increasing knowledge of the side effects of MR imaging further adjustment of the advised limits can be expected.

REFERENCES

1. Adams DF: Biological effect and potential hazards of nuclear magnetic imaging. Cardiovasc Intervent Radiol 8: 260, 1986.

2. Weinreb JC, Maravilla KR, Peshock R, Payne J: Magnetic resonance imaging: Improving patient tolerance and safety. AJR 143: 1285, 1984.

3. New PFL, Rosen BR, Brady TJ, et al.: Potential hazards and artefacts of ferromagnetic and nonferromagnetic surgical and dental materials and devices in nuclear magnetic resonance imaging. Radiology 147: 139, 1983.

4. Finn EJ, Di Chiro G, Brooks RA, Sato S: Ferromagnetic materials in patients: Detection before imaging. Radiology 156: 139, 1985.

5. Bureau of Radiological Health: Guide-lines for evaluating electromagnetic exposure risk for trials and clinical NMR systems. Washington D.C.: Department of Health and Human Services, U.S. Public Health Service, Food and Drug Administration, 1982.

6. Budinger TF: Safety of NMR in vivo imaging and spectroscopy. In: Medical Magnetic Resonance Imaging and Spectroscopy, Budinger TF, Margulis AR (eds.) Society of Magnetic Resonance in Medicine, Berkeley, CA. 1986, 215-233.

7. Pavlicek W, Geisinger M, Castle L, et al.: The effects of nuclear magnetic resonance on patients with cardiac pace-makers. Radiology 147: 149, 1983.

8. Budinger TF, Cullander C: Health effects of in vivo magnetic resonance. In: Clinical Magnetic Resonance Imaging, Margulis AR, Higgins CB, Kaufman L, Crooks LE (eds): Radiological Research and Education Foundation, San Francisco, 1983.

9. Rabinovitch B, Maling JE, Weissblut M: Enzyme substrate reaction in very high magnetic fields. Biophys J. 7: 187, 1967.

10. Nunnally RL, Bottomley PA: Assessment of pharmacological treatment of myocardial infarction by phosphorus-31 NMR with surface coils. Science 211: 177, 1980.

11. Radda GK, Seeley PJ: Recent studies on cellular metabolism by nuclear magnetic resonance. Ann Rev Physiol 41: 749, 1979.

12. Geacintov NE, van Nostrand F, Becker JF, et al.: Magnetic field induced orientation of photosynthetic systems. Biochem Biophys Acta 262: 65, 1972.

13. Murayama M: Orientation of sickled erythrocytes in a magnetic field. Nature 202: 420, 1965.

14. Moore BR: Is the homing pigeon's map geomagnetic? Nature 285: 69, 1980.

15. Gaffey CT, Tenforde TS: Bioelectric properties of frog sciatic nerves

during exposure to static magnetic fields. <u>Radiat Environ Biophys</u> 22: 61, 1983.

16. Liboff RL: Neuromagnetic thresholds. <u>J Theor Biol</u> 83: 427, 1980.

17. d'Arsonval MA: Dispositifs pour la mesure des courants alternatifs a toutes fréquences. <u>CR Soc Biol</u> 3: 451, 1896.

18. Barlow HB, Kohn HI, Walsh EG: The effects of dark adaption and light upon the electric thresholds of the human eye. <u>J Physiol</u> 148: 376, 1947.

19. Budinger TF: Thresholds for physiological effects due to RF and magnetic fields used in NMR imaging. <u>IEEE Trans Nucl Sci NS</u> 26: 2821, 1979.

20. Bore PJ, Galloway GJ, Styles P, et al.: Are quenches dangerous? <u>Magn Res Med</u> 3: 112, 1986.

21. National Radiological Protection Board: Revised guidance on acceptable limits of exposure during nuclear magnetic resonance clinical imaging. <u>Brit Journ Rad</u> 56: 974, 1983.

22. Roy OZ: Summary of cardiac fibrillation thresholds for 60 Hz currents and voltages applied directly to the heart. <u>Med Biol Engineering and Computing</u> 18: 657, 1980.

23. Ueno S, Lovsun P, Oberg A: On the effect of altering magnetic fields on action potential in lobster giant axon. In: <u>Proceedings of the 5th Nordic Meeting on Medical and Biological Engineering</u>, Umea, 1981.

24. Bassett CAL, Pilla AA, Pawluk RJ: A non-operative salvage of surgical resistant pseudarthroses and non-unions by pulsating electromagnetic fields. <u>Clin Orthop</u> 124: 128, 1977.

25. Adair RE, Berglund LG: On the thermoregulatory consequences of NMR imaging. <u>Magn Res Imag</u> 4: 321, 1986.

26. Davis PL, Crooks L, Arakawa M, et al.: Potential hazards in NMR imaging: eating effects of changing magnetic fields and RF fields on small metallic implants. <u>AJR</u> 137: 857, 1981.

27. Mechlin M, Thickman D, Kressel HY, et al.: Magnetic resonance imaging of postoperative patients with metallic implants. <u>AJR</u> 143: 1281, 1984.

28. Laakman RW, Kaufman B, Han JS, et al.: MR imaging in patients with metallic implants. <u>Radiology</u> 157: 711, 1985.

29. Soulen RL, Budinger TF, Higgins CB: Magnetic resonance imaging of prosthetic heart valves. <u>Radiology</u> 154: 705, 1985.

SECTION II NEURO IMAGING

MAGNETIC RESONANCE IMAGING OF THE CENTRAL NERVOUS SYSTEM

G.M. Bydder

INTRODUCTION

The first magnetic resonance imaging (MRI) description of pathological features in the central nervous system was published in 1980 (1). Since that time the technique has progressed rapidly and although progress must inevitably slow down soon, the last year has been as productive as any previous year in terms of technical developments. There are now over 500 MRI machines installed or ordered throughout the world and it is estimated that over 300.000 patients have been studied. The principal area of clinical interest in MRI remains the central nervous system and the development of MRI has obvious parallels with that of X-ray Computed Tomography (CT) although there are also differences. For example, iodinated contrast media were already in clinical use when CT was introduced whereas contrast agents have had to be specifically developed for use with MRI.

The major technical advances have been an improvement in image quality with most manufacturers now using a 256 x 256 reconstruction matrix and some also having available a 512 x 512 reconstruction matrix. More specific improvements have included the use of surface and closely coupled coils and the first clinical trials of Gadolinium-DTPA, a paramagnetic contrast agent. The arguments about the effects of higher field on proton imaging are not resolved but higher fields have made chemical shift and sodium imaging easier.

The costs of MRI machines have increased with the general trend towards high field imaging, although this trend is not being followed by some Japanese manufacturers, nor by one Finnish group (Instrumentarium) who have produced an almost portable MRI machine operating at less than one twentieth of the industry 'standard' (i.e. 0.02 Tesla versus 0.5 Tesla).

There are several general reviews of MR imaging in the CNS available (2,3,4) which provide a useful introduction to the subject.

PARAMAGNETIC CONTRAST AGENTS

Most of the soft tissue contrast apparent in MR images is a result of differences in the tissue relaxation times T_1 and T_2. Paramagnetic contrast agents offer the possibility of changing tissue T_1 and T_2. They usually contain unpaired electrons within the metallic ions manganese, gadolinium or iron - the metallic ions are chelated in order to reduce their toxicity. The first such compound used in clinical practice has been Gadolinium-DTPA produced by Schering (5). It is injected intravenously and circulates in the vascular system after which it is excreted unchanged through the kidneys. Like iodinated contrast media it only crosses the abnormal blood-brain-barrier. It then produces a decrease in T_1 and T_2. Its most important applications have been in enhancing benign tumors and demonstrating the margin between tumor and edema in malignant tumors (6).

DEMYELINATING DISEASE

Multiple sclerosis was the disease in which an advantage for MRI over existing techniques was first demonstrated; it is also the disease par excellence in which MRI has reached the stage of a routine application. The study of patients with suspected MS is now 'bread and butter' MRI. With wider experience a range of normal variants and 'traps' in diagnosing this disease are now being recognised. Small areas of increased signal intensity may be seen as a normal finding at the anterolateral angles of the lateral ventricles with spin-echo images, and the body and tail of the caudate nucleus may be confused with MS lesions.

The sensitivity of MRI in multiple sclerosis is high but the findings are relatively non-specific and similar or identical features may be seen in other demyelinating diseases as well as vascular disease, SLE, sarcoidosis, some infective conditions, periventricular edema and other conditions although some distinction is possible in individual cases. Nevertheless the principal advantage of MRI is that it demonstrates lesions in clinically silent areas of the brain and this is important in patients whose symptoms or signs are minimal. It is impossible to say with absolute certainty that a patient has not got MS, but a negative examination with the most sensitive imaging technique available is certainly significant.

Studies have been performed comparing the sensitivity of different pulse sequences in MS (7,8). In general, appropriate spin-echo sequences are better than inversion recovery sequences in most areas except the brainstem.

Contrast enhancement has also been demonstrated in some lesions with Gadolinium-DTPA but it remains to be seen whether or not the diagnostic yield will be increased in MS with MRI to the degree it has been with double dose and delayed contrast enhancement with X-ray CT.

Chemical shift imaging has been suggested as a technique for detecting denatured lipid in demyelinating disease in order to improve specificity but no results are available as yet.

A problem which has arisen, as a result of the general trend towards higher field MRI, has been difficulty in obtaining spin echo sequences with high T_2 dependence in which the signal from CSF is less than that from brain. This has arisen as a result of the fact that the T_1 of brain increases with magnetic field more than that of CSF. It is therefore difficult to allow the brain to recover its magnetisation while choosing a repetition rate of scanning sufficient to prevent the CSF from recovery. When the signal from CSF is less than brain, lesions (which are highlighted) cannot be confused with partial volume effects between brain and CSF; this is not the case when the CSF signal is greater than brain.

The appearances in a range of other demyelinating diseases are now being described, and while many of these have much in common with MS, others such as the leucodystrophies display confluent patterns or may display disease largely confined to white matter tracts as with post-infectious demyelinating disease (Fig. 1).

CEREBROVASCULAR DISEASE

Much wider experience has been obtained in imaging cerebro-vascular disease. The most important additional observations concern intracranial hemorrhage which has been studied in detail by Gomori et al (9). Whilst earlier reports drew attention to the decreased T_1 in hematoma several days after the ictus, more detailed studies have demonstrated an earlier phase in which both T_1 and T_2 are prolonged. The T_1 may then shorten and after a period of days to weeks, increase again. The mechanism for this change is not fully understood but it has been suggested that free ferric ion, deoxyhemoglobin or methemoglobin may produce the change as a consequence of their paramagnetic activity. From a clinical point of view, difficulty has been reported in recognising hemorrhage in the acute or

30

subacute phase. On the other hand, in late phases of hemorrhage characteristic features may be observed which enable hemorrhage to be distinguished from other space occupying lesions in cases where there is doubt on CT (10).

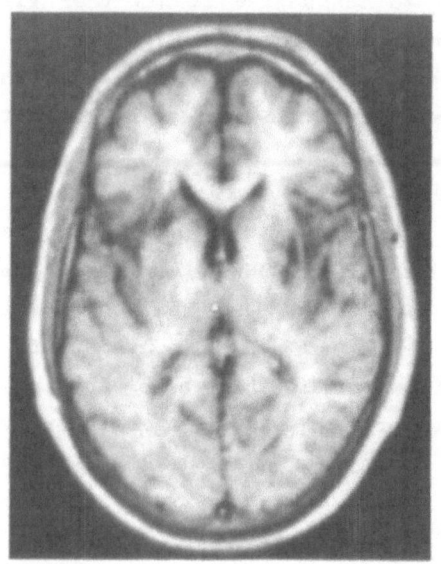 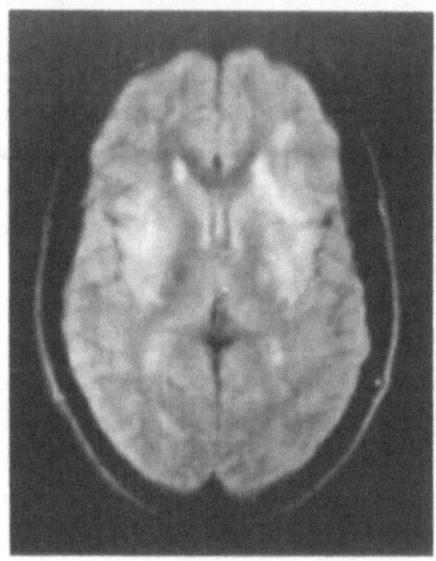

FIGURE 1.   Postinfectious demyelinating disease: a) IR1500/500/44 and b) SE1500/80 scans. Most of the change is seen within white matter.

Cerebral infarction in the brainstem is more readily recognised with MRI than with CT and there is a suggestion from experimental results that the early phases of infarction may also be more readily recognized.

Periventricular lesions are a frequent observation in the elderly (11) and it is thought that these may well represent subclinical infarction.

It is possible to quantify blood flow with MRI (12,13) and this may have a role in the study of vessels inaccessible to Doppler techniques, such as the basilar artery. There is also considerable interest in developing techniques for the study of tissue perfusion (14).

The paramagnetic contrast agent Gd-DTPA has been used in a limited range of cerebrovascular disease. In general terms the results parallel those seen with X-ray CT however, flow effects in aneurysms and arterio-venous malformations may be so marked that the effect of contrast enhancement, that would be expected by analogy with CT, is minimal or absent. On the other hand calcification may obscure contrast enhancement on CT scans and this may be obvious with MRI.

CENTRAL NERVOUS SYSTEM INFECTION

Most early MR imaging systems were installed in factories, laboratories or other clinically inaccessible sites which made the study of seriously ill patients difficult. As a result studies of infectious disease have been limited and then largely confined to chronic conditions in which the patient's condition was stable.

It is clear that MRI is sensitive to abnormality and this may be focal or generalized. The changes in the temporal lobes are well demonstrated in Herpes simplex encephalitis. Less specific changes are seen in other generalised infections. Often the changes are in a periventricular distribution and while the appearances are defintely abnormal, they may be quite non specific.

Abscesses are well displayed but so far no specific features have been identified to separate them from similar mass lesions. Associated calcification is poorly seen.

An interesting observation has been the pial-ependymal-line, a track extending from the pia to the ependyma in some cases of infective disease (15). The exact etiology and significance of this feature remains uncertain.

As with other diseases in the brain, contrast agents are likely to increase diagnostic specificity.

BENIGN TUMORS

Meningioma: Two reports have appeared indicating that meningiomas are less satisfactorily seen with unenhanced MRI than they are with contrast enhanced CT (3,4). This is an important finding because meningiomas are amongst the most treatable of tumors and are well demonstrated and diagnosed with a high level of accuracy using enhanced CT. They have a wide variety of presentations so that an MRI screening technique must be able to detect them with a high level of certainty. The most commonly used screening examination in MRI has involved the use of highly T_2 dependent spin echo sequences. Unfortunately some meningiomas do not display an increase in T_2 so tumors may then need to be detected by their indirect signs.

32

The inversion recovery sequence is more sensitive than spin echo in detecting meningiomas and is also highly sensitive to contrast enhancement. In our own experience using inversion recovery and contrast enhancement the results in meningioma have been equal to or better than those of CT (although 3 of the 15 cases studied only had second generation CT scans).

Acoustic Neuroma: The lack of signal from the petrous temporal bone provides the setting for the detection of acoustic neuromas with MRI. The normal internal auditory canal is seen without difficulty and soft tissue may be detected within the canal or cerebellopontine angle with spin echo sequences. Acoustic neuromas show variable appearances with a significant minority not displaying an increase in T_2. We have so far demonstrated 43 acoustic neuromas. No case shown with CT or CT cisternography was not shown with MRI and 5 additional cases were demonstrated. These included two with negative air-CT cisternograms. It seems possible therefore that MRI can be used for diagnosis of both large and small acoustic neuromas.

Contrast enhancement was seen in all 13 cases in which it was used (Fig. 2) but only provided additional new diagnostic information in one patient with a small intracanalicular tumor and a second with a recurrence.

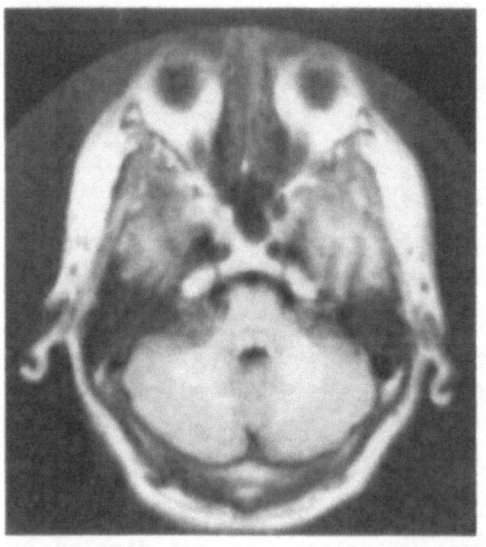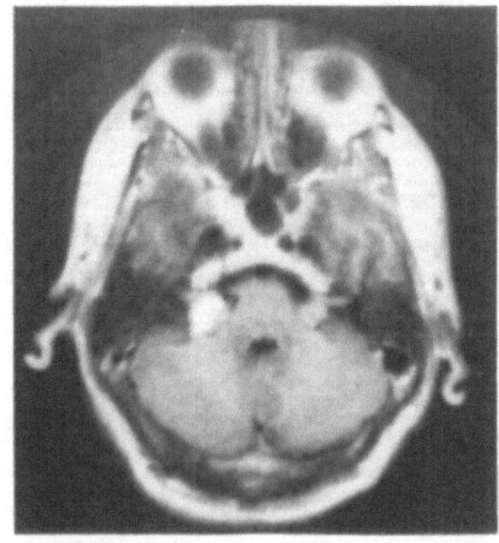

FIGURE 2. Bilateral acoustic neuroma: a) before and b) after I.V. Gd-DTPA: IR1500/500/44 scans. Both tumors are better seen in (b).

Pituitary Tumors: MRI has shown a similar level of accuracy to CT in detection of pituitary tumors. Direct sagittal and coronal imaging is easier with MRI (Fig. 3) but there are difficulties in resolving small tumors. Determining the extent of large tumors is relatively straightforward.

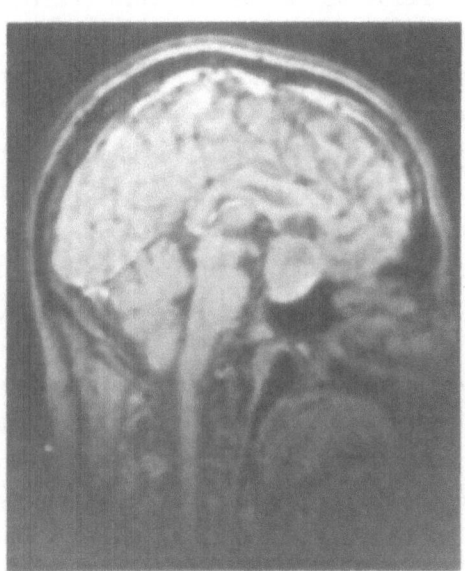 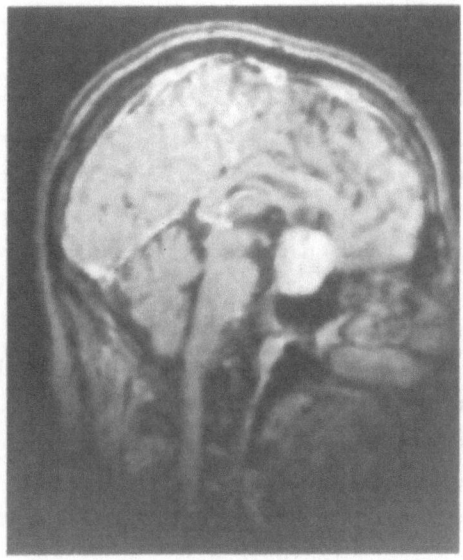

FIGURE 3. Pituitary adenoma: a) before and b) after I.V. Gd-DTPA. Enhancement is seen within the tumor.

Other Benign Tumors: Lipomas have a characteristic appearance as a result of their short T_1. Any associated calcification is poorly seen but the midline plane lends itself to direct sagittal imaging and this has proved satisfactory so far. CT also shows specific features and demonstrates calcification as well.

Craniopharyngiomas are likewise well displayed, using direct sagittal and coronal imaging.

MALIGNANT TUMORS

Damadian initially drew attention to the increased T_1 and T_2 of animal tumors in 1971 and this change in relaxation time is a notable feature in most malignant tumors. However in a later paper (16) Damadian also noted that one type of tumor (malignant melanoma) did not always display an increase in T_1 and T_2. Since that time the initial observation of increased relaxation times of tumors has been confirmed repeatedly; but also the number of exceptions has also increased (17).

As with benign tumors, the most important recent development has been the use of intravenous Gadolinium-DTPA. Prior to the use of this contrast agent differentiation between tumor and edema was a disadvantage of MRI in relation to contrast enhanced CT, but better results have now been achieved with MRI. In 4 of 17 malignant tumors studied with MRI areas of apparent 'edema' seen with contrast enhanced CT and unenhanced MRI displayed contrast enhancement and therefore probably were areas of tumor infiltration (18). From experience with stereotactic CT biopsy it is likely that tumor is infiltrating outside the rim of enhancement seen with MRI. Nevertheless defining the bulk of the tumor is valuable for biopsy and radiotherapy, as well as surgery.

Systems for stereotactic biopsy have now been developed for MRI (19) and used in clinical practice (20). Only relatively minor modifications are necessary to systems already used with CT. Ferromagnetic materials must be avoided, as must closed conducting loops which may permit cirulating eddy currents. MRI sensitive materials must be used as the coordinate indicators.

Whilst the advantages of MRI in imaging tumors in the posterior fossa were recognised early in the development of this technique (21,22) MRI also has advantages in the supratentorial region. In these cases CT is not generally negative, but only shows a mass effect or hydrocephalus without indicating the actual site of the lesion. We have now studied 16 cases in this category and in 14 cases the MRI scan was able to display more specific information about the size and site of the tumor. This included some benign tumors (Colloid cyst, meningioma) as well as malignant tumors.

Malignant melanoma is of considerable theoretical interest as a tumor which consistently displays a pattern of decrease in T_1 rather than the usual increase (Fig. 4) but this pattern may also be seen in patients treated with radiotherapy, some benign tumors, and some hemorrhagic tumors.

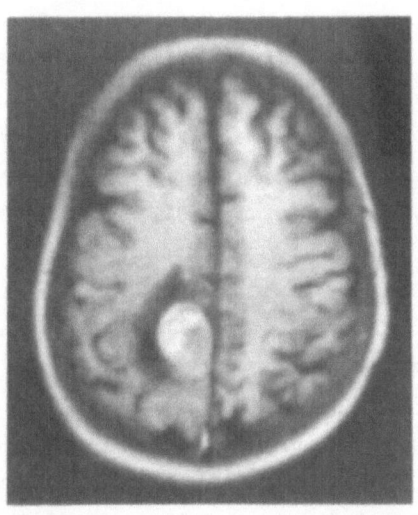

FIGURE 4.   Malignant melanoma metastasis: IR1500/500/44 scan.   The tumor
has a high signal intensity.

DEGENERATIVE DISEASE
   The general features of atrophic disease parallel those seen with X-ray
CT. A greater degree of abnormality is seen in Wilson's Disease (23, Fig.
12) and findings similar to CT are seen in Huntington's Disease. Atrophy
of the substantia migra has been identified in Parkinson's Disease. Late
atrophic features are seen in a variety of heredo-familial disorders.

PEDIATRICS
   Pediatric MRI requires a number of modifications of technique.
Although general anesthesia is clearly justified in serious illness it is
not possible to justify it for infants and children with relatively minor
disease or for normal controls, so that a system of oral sedation is
necessary if a wide variety of disease is being studied. We do not sedate
children during the first 3-6 months of life. We use oral sedation up to
about 4-6 years and beyond this age do not use sedation but place a member
of staff in the machine with the child to provide 'entertainment'.
   We have found spherical coils matched to the child's size a
considerable improvement over conventional saddle designs (24). These are
constructed in a range of 10 sizes and the child is fitted with one

36

immediately prior to the examination.

The water content of the brain in neonates is 92-95% and drops to 82-85% in the first two years of life. The increased water content is accompanied by a 200-300% increase of relaxation times. Image sequences require adjustment for these large changes in order to show satisfactory contrast with the time parameters for all sequences requiring an increase.

· Another feature of note about the neonatal brain is the normal process of myelination which occurs particularly during the first two years of life but continues into the second decade. This is readily demonstrated with inversion recovery sequences and delays or deficits in this process have been reported (25).

A range of vascular, ischaemic, and anoxic changes have been observed including hemorrhage (Fig. 5), infarction, periventricular leukomalacia and anoxic ischemic encephalopathy. Follow up of these patients has been possible.

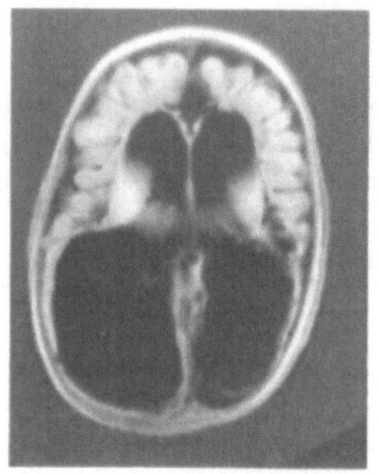 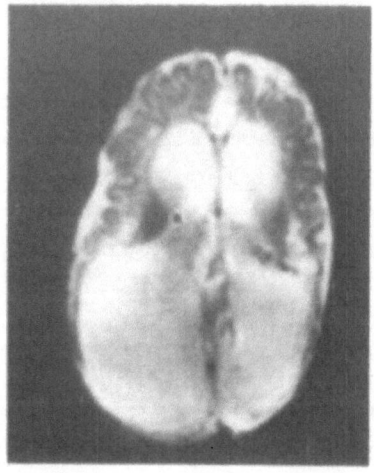

FIGURE 5. Infant aged 8 months: Hydrocephalus and bilateral thalamic hemorrhage: a) IR1800/600/44 and b) PS1660/193 scans. The ventricles are dilated. High signal is seen in the thalamus in (a) and low signal is seen in (b).

Hydrocephalus and periventricular edema are readily observed. Ventricular shunts produce a local deficit but most of the image is still adequate in quality.

Pediatric tumors are also well demonstrated (26). Although the spectrum
of disease differs from that in adults the essential features in both
benign and malignant tumors are similar. It is possible that tumors in the
first years of life may appear different relative to the surrounding brain
(because of the increased relaxation time of the normal brain) but our
experience in this area is limited.

CONCLUSION

MRI is still evolving rapidly and there are many other technical
developments which have already passed the laboratory phase and are
awaiting clinical evaluation.

Decrease in the normal slice thickness of 7-10mm to 2-3mm has been
achieved by most manufacturers and appears likely to be of particular
value in lesions around the third ventricle and in the cervical cord.

Sodium imaging is available at high field (27) and the early results
suggest high sensitivity in detecting edema and infarction.

There are many other applications of paramagnetic contrast agents yet
to be studied including demyelinating disease and cerebrovascular disease.

Chemical shift imaging which enables fat and lipid to be separated
appears promising as a method of adding specificity to MRI diagnosis; it
may also be of value in identifying specific metabolites. The most
important use to date has been elimination of the signal from bone marrow.

MR spectroscopy is also being developed and while no major clinical
application has yet been demonstrated its potential remains high.

While the technical improvements in MRI over the last three years have
been remarkable, major questions remain about the cost of installing and
running such equipment. The trend to high field and the interest in
spectroscopy (which requires a high field) has resulted in a considerable
increase in the price of already expensive machines. Early in the
development of MRI one of the research objectives was a good quality
imaging machine of realistic price for service use. This may come back
into fashion, but at the moment this objective is low in most
manufacturers' priorities. Yet the information that is available on the
economics of the present range of MRI machines indicates that they are
more expensive to install and run than CT machines, and that cost
effectiveness is only likely to be achieved with very considerable effort.

REFERENCES

1. Hawkes RC, Holland GN, Moore WS, et al: Nuclear magnetic resonance (NMR) tomography of the brain: A preliminary clinical assessment with demonstration of pathology. J Comput Assist Tomogr 4: 577-586, 1980

2. Brant-Zawadzki M, Davis PL, Crooks LE, et al: NMR demonstration of cerebral abnormalities: Comparison with CT. AJR 140: 847-854, 1983

3. Zimmerman RD, Bilaniuk LT, Goldberg HL, et al: Cerebral nuclear magnetic resonance imaging: Early results with a 0.12 T resistive system. AJR 141: 1187-1193, 1983

4. Bradley WG, Waluch V, Yadley RA, et al: Comparison of CT and NMR in 400 cases of the brain and cervical cord. Radiology 152: 695-702, 1984

5. Weinmann H-J, Brasch RC, Press WR, et al: Characterics of gadolinium-DTPA complex. AJR 142: 619-624, 1984

6. Carr DH, Brown J, Bydder GM, et al: Clinical use of intravenous gadolinium-DTPA as a contrast agent in NMR imaging of cerebral tumours. Lancet i: 484-486, 1984

7. Runge VM, Price AC, Kirschner HS, Allen JH, Partain CL, James AE: Magnetic resonance imaging of multiple sclerosis: a study of pulse-technique efficacy. AJNR 5: 691-702, 1984

8. Young IR, Randell CP, Kaplan PE, et al: Nuclear magnetic imaging in white matter disease of the brain using spin-echo sequences. J Comput Assist Tomogr 7: 290-294, 1983

9. Gomori J, Grossman RI, Goldberg HI, et al: Intracranial hematomas: imaging by high field MR. Radiology 57: 87-93, 1985

10. Bailes DR, Young IR, Thomas DJ, et al: NMR imaging of the brain using spin-echo sequences. Clin Rad 33: 395-414, 1982

11. Bradley WG, Waluch V, Brant-Zawadzki M, et al: Patchy periventricular white matter lesions in the elderly: A common observation during NMR imaging. Non-Invasive Imaging 1: 35-42, 1984

12. Crooks LE, Kaufman L: NMR imaging of blood flow. Br Med Bull 40: 167-169, 1984

13. Bryant DJ, Payne JA, Firmin D, Longmore DB: Measurement of flow with NMR imaging using a gradient pulse and phase difference technique. J Comput Assist Tomogr 8(4): 588-593, 1984

14. Le Bihan D, Breton E, Lallenad D: Evaluation of diffusion and perfusion using MR imaging of IVIM. Radiology 161: 368, 1986

15. Davidson HD, Steiner RE: MRI of infections of the central nervous

system. AJNR 6: 499-504, 1985

16. Damadian R, Zaner K, Hor D: Brain tumors by NMR. Physiol Chem Phys 5: 381-402, 1983

17. MacKay IM, Bydder GM, Young IR: Magnetic resonance imaging of central nervous system tumors which do not display evidence of an increase in T_1 or T_2. J Comput Assist Tomogr 9(6): 1055-1061, 1985

18. Graif M, Bydder GM, Steiner RE, Neindorf HP, Thomas DG, Young IR: Contrast enhanced MRI of malignant brain tumors. AJNR 6: 855-862, 1985

19. Leksell L, Leksell D, Schwebel J: Stereotaxis and nuclear magnetic resonance. J Neurol Neurosurg Psych 48: 14-18, 1985

20. Thomas DGT, Davis CH, Ingram S, Olney JS, Bydder GM, Young IR: Stereotactic biopsy of the brain under magnetic resonance imaging control. AJNR 7: 161-163, 1986

21. McGinnis BD, Brady TJ, New PFJ et al: Nuclear magnetic resonance (NMR) imaging of tumours in the posterior fossa. J Comput Assist Tomogr 7: 575-584, 1983

22. Randell CP, Collins AG, Hayward R, et al: NMR imaging of the posterior fossa tumours. AJR 141: 489-496, 1983

23. Lawler GA, Pennock JM, Steiner RE, et al: NMR imaging in Wilson's Disease. J Comput Assist Tomogr 7: 1-8, 1983

24. Bydder GM, Butsen PR, Harman RR, Gilderdale DJ, Young IR: Use of spherical receiver coils in magnetic resonance imaging of the brain. J Comput Assist Tomogr 9(2): 413-414, 1985

25. Johnson MA, Pennock JM, Bydder GM, et al: Clinical NMR imaging of the brain in children: Normal and neurologic disease. AJNR 4: 1013-1026, 1983

26. Peterman SD, Steiner RE, Byddor CM: NMR imaging of intracranial tumors in children and adolescents. AJNR 5(6): 703-709, 1984

27. Hilal SK, Maudsley AA, Ra JB, et al: In vivo NMR imaging of sodium-23 in the human head. J Comput Assist Tomogr 9: 1-7, 1985

CONTRAST AGENTS IN MRI: CLINICAL APPLICATIONS OF GADOLINIUM-DTPA IN THE CENTRAL NERVOUS SYSTEM

A. DE ROOS, D. BALERIAUX

INTRODUCTION
   Gadolinium-diethylene-triamine-penta-acetic acid
(Gd-DTPA/dimeglumine) is a clinically useful paramagnetic contrast agent for magnetic resonance imaging (MRI) (1-4). Due to its favorable pharmacokinetic properties and lack of adverse reactions Gd-DTPA proved to be safe for use in humans. When subtle or no differences in signal intensity between normal and pathological tissue exist, Gd-DTPA can enhance contrast between abnormal and normal tissue, thereby increasing sensitivity and specificity of the study. Gd-DTPA produces local alterations in the magnetic environment that enhance MR-relaxation of protons. Unlike conventional radiographic contrast agents that are directly visualized, Gd-DTPA is imaged indirectly by enhancement of proton relaxation due to the seven unpaired electrons of the Gd-ion, which determine the paramagnetic strength.
   Both shortening of T1 relaxation time and prolongation of T2 relaxation time will increase MR signal intensity. The longitudinal (T1) and transverse (T2) relaxation times are decreased by Gd-DTPA. Gd-DTPA (in the usual dose of 0.1 mmol per kg body weight) will increase the signal intensity of tissues perfused by this contrast agent, in T1 weighted images. Thus, Gd-DTPA permits the use of shorter TR and TE, thereby shortening the imaging time and it may obviate time-consuming T2 weighted pulse sequences. However, depending on the concentration of Gd-DTPA, shortening in T2 relaxation time can decrease signal intensity, as opposed to an increase of signal intensity based on decrease of T1 relaxation time (11). Depending on perfusion and vascularity there is a rapid distribution of Gd-DTPA limited to the extracellular compartment of the body. Therefore, Gd-DTPA can be used as a marker of organ perfusion, renal function, thus identifying inflammatory lesions, viable tumor, and disruption of the blood-brain barrier. Gd-DTPA is excreted primarily by glomerular filtration with a short half-life time. The initial distribution of Gd-DTPA is related to blood flow and tissue perfusion and causes strong effects on signal intensity in the first several minutes. However, in diseased tissue, there can be an altered perfusion and distribution of Gd-DTPA, causing better contrast enhancement at a later moment in time. For example, a longer diffusion time of Gd-DTPA into an area of necrosis can make it necessary to wait for a certain period to optimize contrast enhancement. On the other hand, it can be necessary to use fast imaging techniques to detect differences in signal intensity when critical time-dependent changes occur immediately after injection of Gd-DTPA.

TECHNICAL CONSIDERATIONS
   Spin-echo technique
Since the influence of the presence of Gd-DTPA --at the usual dosage of 0.1 mmol per kg body weight-- is usually more strongly affecting T1 than T2 (15), T1 weighted images (for instance obtained by the Spin Echo pulse sequence with TR = 500 ms and TE = 30 ms (SE 500/30)) are appropriate for the detection of Gd-DTPA induced signal intensity changes. In the following section a numerical example of the signal intensity changes after

Gd-DTPA administration is given.
   In a tissue with typical T1 and T2 values of 500 ms and 70 ms respectively, application of an SE 500/30 pulse sequence will result in a signal
intensity of 0.41 (arbitrary units). This value is obtained from the
approximative equation for SE signal intensity (Int):

$$Int = C \cdot [1-exp(-TR/T1)].exp(-TE/T2)$$

When T1 and T2 both increase or decrease, the effect of this change on the
signal intensity is partially cancelled. A decrease of 10% in both T1 and
T2 would hardly be noticed. The signal intensity would only raise from
0.41 to 0.42.
   However, if we assume a 50% decrease in T1 and a 25% decrease in T2 value of the tissue under investigation after Gd-DTPA injection (T1=250 ms,
T2=53 ms), the SE 500/30 pulse sequence would result in a signal intensity
of 0.49. Thus, the injection of contrast agent would in this case cause an
18% increase in signal intensity. It is not exactly known how much the
T1 and T2 values in-vivo are changed by Gd-DTPA, but the example above
gives a general understanding of the effect of Gd-DTPA.

   Fast-field-echo imaging
   In fast field echo (FFE) imaging the RF pulse angle value is an additional factor influencing the signal intensity (14). The equation above
describes only the effect of T1, T2, TR and TE on the SE signal intensity.
In FFE imaging T2* has to be considered in stead of T2, since the FFE sequence uses a gradient echo which does not correct for field inhomogeneities (T2* is the apparent T2 value, which includes the influence of field
inhomogeneities).The equation

$$Int = \frac{C \cdot (sinA).[1-exp(-TR/T1)].exp(-TE/T2^*)}{1-cosA.exp(-TR/T1)}$$

gives a first order approximation of the signal intensities obtained using
a reduced RF pulse angle of the value A.
   Reduction of the pulse angle allows the application of a smaller TR value without the loss of too much signal due to saturation. The pulse angle
yielding maximum signal varies with the value of T1/TR. It is possible to
make several images during the wash-in phase of a contrast agent, in a way
analogous to dynamic CT scanning.
   For most tissues a pulse angle of about 40 degrees in combination with a
TR of 50 ms will give the maximum signal intensity. However, using this
combination of pulse angle and TR,. one obtains an image with only little
intensity difference between the various tissues. This may be explained as
follows: in most human tissues T1 and T2 values appear to be 'coupled',
i.e. an increase in T1 is usually accompanied by an increase in T2. Using
a pulse angle of approximately 10 degrees, the T1 dependency of the signal
intensity will be minimized. The signal intensity thus obtained is not the
maximum possible, but now intensity differences between tissues will appear as a consequence of T2 differences. Application of a large pulse
angle of e.g. 90 or 120 degrees results in a T1 weighted image (9).
   The influence of Gd-DTPA on the signal intensity of FFE images is similar to its effects on SE images. Since the T1 value is more strongly affected than the T2 value, the effect of Gd on FFE images will also be
better observed in the more T1 weighted images. The following example gi-

ves some insight into this matter: Tissue parameters are for instance T1 = 500 ms, T2* = 30 ms. In an image obtained with an FFE pulse sequence with TR = 50 ms and TE = 13 ms, this tissue would show signal intensities of 0.10, 0.13 and 0.06 at pulse angles of 10, 40 and 90 degrees, respectively. Assuming again a 50% decrease of T1 and a 25% decrease of T2* after Gd-DTPA administration, the same tissue would show up with signal intensities of 0.09, 0.18 and 0.10, i.e. a change of -10%, 38% and 67% as compared to the pre-contrast images, respectively. Thus, the effect of Gd will be best observed in the more T1 weighted FFE-pulse sequences.

CLINICAL APPLICATIONS IN THE CENTRAL NERVOUS SYSTEM

Gd-DTPA-enhanced MRI was initially applied to study the extension of brain tumors (5-8, 10, 12, 13, 15-18). Especially, differentiation of tumor tissue from perifocal edema in patients with glioblastomas and metastases can be difficult without the administration of Gd-DTPA. Even T2 weighted images can be inaccurate to delineate tumor from perifocal edema with sufficient differences in contrast. After administration of Gd-DTPA the signal intensity of viable tumor increases and no change is observed in signal intensity of perifocal edema providing optimal demarcation of tumor. The contrast agent demonstrates disruption of the blood-brain barrier and perfusion of viable tumor tissue (Fig. 1).

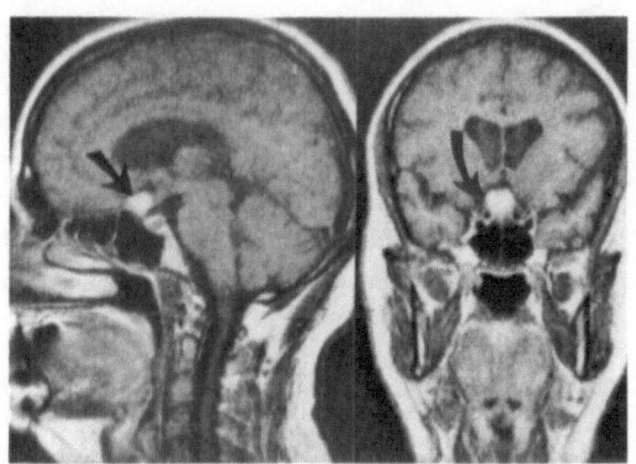

FIGURE 1. a) Sagittal T1-weighted MR image
demonstrates enhancement of meningioma (arrow) after Gadolinium injection. Before contrast administration tumor appeared as isointense and was difficult to delineate.

b) Coronal T1-weighted MR image
shows relation of enhancing meningioma (arrow) to surrounding structures.

Tumors are best visualized in the first minutes after injection of the contrast agent. Necrotic tumor demonstrates a delayed wash-in of the contrast agent as compared to viable tumor tissue.

Intracanalicular acoustic neuromas and meningiomas may appear isointense as compared to surrounding tissue on both T1 and T2 weighted images. Therefore, enhancement after Gd-DTPA injection of these lesions will improve diagnostic specificity (7). Contrast enhancement of nasal mucosa, pituitary gland, cavernous sinus, cavernous portions of cranial nerves, and choroid plexus is a normal occurence and can be applied to evaluate effective contrast injection (13). In a blind multi-reader evaluation, Gd-DTPA-enhanced MRI proved to increase diagnostic specificity and overall confidence in border definition of metastasis and meningiomas. In general, Gd-DTPA-enhanced scans improved diagnostic accuracy in establishing the correct diagnosis (Fig. 2).

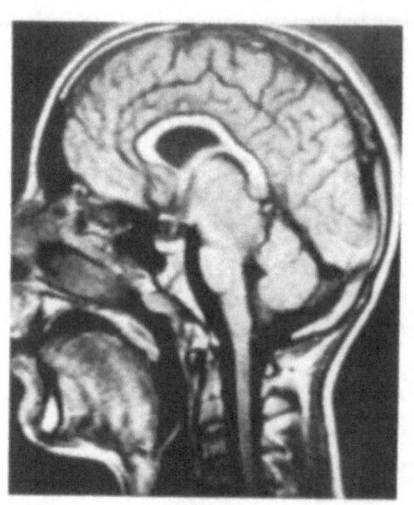 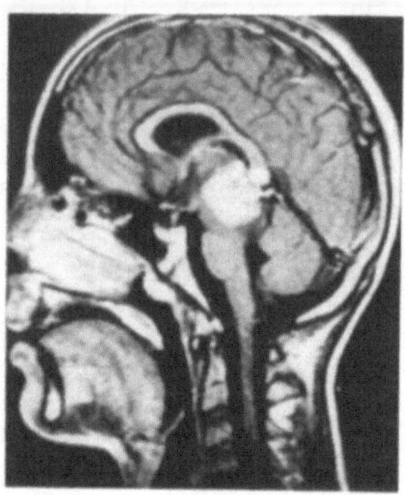

FIGURE 2   a) Sagittal MR images through a pinealioma invading the brain
              stem.
              Sagittal, pre-contrast, SE 400/30. Larger tumor invading
              brain stem is not well delineated.

           b) Sagittal, post-contrast, SE 400/30.
              Marked tumor enhancement is observed. Note extension of tumor
              into corpus callosum, improving diagnostic accuracy.

In patients with multiple sclerosis Gd-enhanced MRI appears to have the ability to separate active from inactive lesions (12). Enhancement of recent plaques is a sensitive marker of disruption of the blood-brain barrier. Some of these enhancing lesions appear to have a high correlation with clinical symptoms.

Although MRI is the optimal imaging modality to diagnose tumors of the spinal cord, precise delineation of tumor extension may be difficult. The use of intravenous injection of Gd-DTPA is extremely valuable in order to demonstrate tumor margins (1, 4) (Fig. 3).

Contrary to low-grade astrocytomas in the brain, low-grade astrocytomas located in the spinal cord show contrast enhancement after gadolinium administration (Fig. 4).

Fast field echo imaging in combination with injection of Gd-DTPA can demonstrate tumor enhancement and temporal uptake of gadolinium can be followed. Gd-DTPA-enhanced MR imaging will probably become a prerequisite for thorough evaluation of spinal tumors.

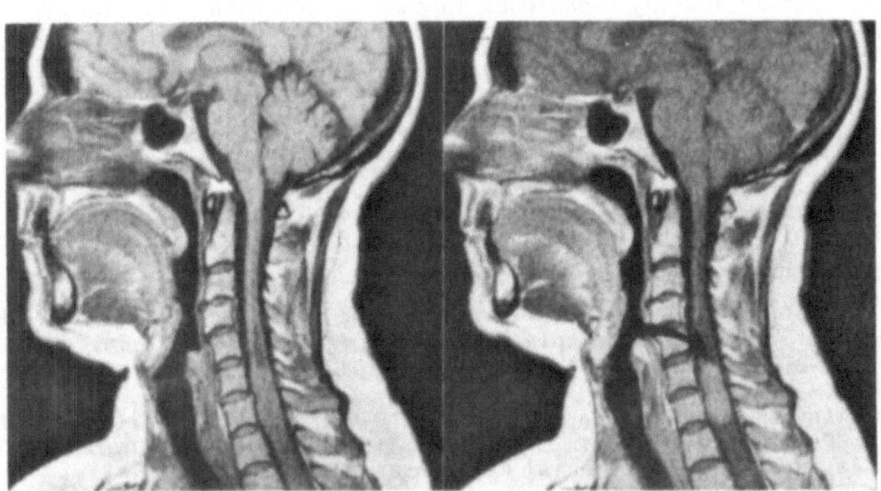

FIGURE 3 a) Sagittal T1-weighted MR image
demonstrates enlargement of cervical myelum with central cavity.

b) After Gadolinium injection tumor demonstrates high signal
intensity (arrow).

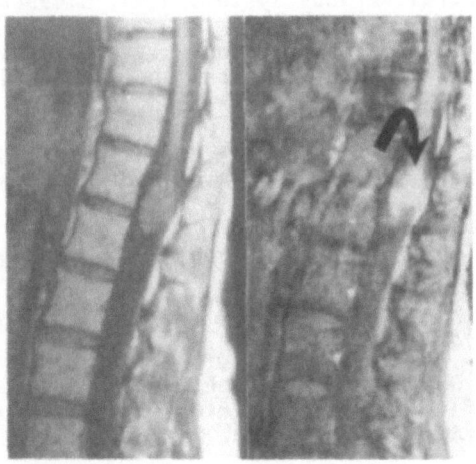

FIGURE 4 a) Sagittal T1-weighted image
clearly demonstrates spinal tumor.

b) Fast scan after injection of Gadolinium shows tumor enhancement (arrow).

REFERENCES

1. Baleriaux, D., Segebarth, C., van Dam, R., Niendorf, H.-P. (1986): Use of fast MR imaging techniques in combination with intravenous injection of Gd-DTPA for the study of spinal cord tumors. Radiology, 161(P):252.

2. Berry, I., Brant-Zawadzki, M., Osaki, L., Brasch, R., Murovic, J., Newton, T.H. (1986): Gd-DTPA in Clinical MR of the Brain: 2. Extraaxial Lesions and Normal Structures. AJNR, 7:789-793.

3. Brant-Zawadzki, M., Berry, I., Osaki, L., Brasch, R., Murovic, J., Norman, D. (1986): Gd-DTPA in Clinical MR of the Brain: 1. Intraaxial Lesions. AJNR, 7:781-788.

4. Bydder, G.M., Brown, J., Niendorf, H.-P., Young, R.I. (1985): Enhancement of Cervical Intraspinal Tumors in MR Imaging with Intravenous Gadolinium-DTPA. J. Comput. Assist. Tomogr., 9(5):847-851.

5. Claussen, C., Laniado, M., Schörner, W., Niendorf, H.-P., Weinmann, H.J., Fiegler, W., Felix, R. (1985): Gadolinium-DTPA in MR Imaging of Glioblastomas and Intracranial Metastases. AJNR, 6:669-674.

6. Claussen, C., Laniado, M., Kazner, E., Schörner, W., Felix, R. (1985): Application of contrast agents in CT and MRI (NMR): their potential in imaging of brain tumors. Neuroradiology, 27:164-171.

7. Curatti, W.L., Graif, M., Kingsley, D.P.E., Niendorf, H.-P., Young, I.R. (1986): Acoustic Neuromas: Gd-DTPA Enhancement in MR Imaging. Radiology, 158:447-451.

8. Davidson, H.D., Steiner, R.E. (1985): Magnetic Resonance Imaging in Infections of the Central Nervous System. AJNR, 6:499-504.

9. Edelman, R.R., Hahn, P.F., Buxton, R., et al. (1986): Rapid MR imaging with suspended respiration: Clinical application in the liver. Radiology, 161:125-131.

10. Felix, R., Schörner, W., Laniado, M., Niendorf, H.-P., Claussen, C., Fiegler, W., Speck, U. (1985): Brain Tumors: MR Imaging with Gadolinium-DTPA. Radiology, 156:681-688.

11. Gadian, D.G., Payne, J.A., Bryant, D.J., Young, I.R., Carr, D.H., Bydder, G.M. (1985): Gadolinium-DTPA as a Contrast Agent in MR Imaging Theoretical Projections and Practical Observations. J. Comput. Assist. Tomogr., 9(2):242-251.

12. Grossman, R.I., Gonzalez-Scarano, F., Atlas, S.W., Galetta, S., Silberberg, D.H. (1986): Multiple Sclerosis: Gadolinium enhancement in MR imaging. Radiology, 161:721-725.

13. van der Meulen, P., Groen, J.P., Cuppen, J.J.M. (1985): Very fast MR imaging by field echoes and small angle excitation. Magn. Reson. Imaging, 3: 297-299.

14. Niendorf, H.-P., Felix, R., Laniado, M., Schörner, W., Claussen, C., Weinmann, H.J. (1985): Gadolinium-DTPA: A New Contrast Agent for Magnetic Resonance Imaging. Radiation Medicine, Vol.3 No.1:7-12.

15. Runge, V.M., Clanton, J.A., Price, A.C., et al. (1985): The use of Gd-DTPA as aperfusion agent and a marker of blood-brain barrier disruption. Magn. Reson. Imaging, 3:43-55.

16. Schörner, W., Laniado, M., Niendorf, H.-P., Schubert, Chr., Felix, R. (1986): Time-dependent changes in image contrast in brain tumors after gadolinium-DTPA. AJNR 7, 1013-1020.

17. Virapongse, C., Mancuso, A., Quisling, R. (1986): Human Brain infarcts: Gd-DTPA-enhanced MR imaging. Radiology, 161:785-794.

SUSPECTED DISEASE OF THE BRAIN – MRI OR CT ?

W. Heindel, W. Steinbrich

This general question is difficult to answer, because the answer will depend on the kind of pathology. However, the try of a general assessment may be allowed just in the beginning: if you look at all pathologies detectable by Magnetic Resonance Imaging (MRI) or Computed Tomography (CT), MRI has demonstrated unequivocally a higher sensitivity. This high sensitivity is due to its higher soft tissue differentiation largely independent of the kind of lesion. On the other hand, the diagnostic specifity of MRI is as good or as bad as that of CT. Thus, MRI should be the primary modality for the initial evaluation of patients with symptoms and/or signs referable to the central nervous system.

MATERIALS AND METHODS

At our institution comparative brain studies have had priority since installation of MR in 1984. We tried to determine the advantages and disadvantages of both procedures by an objective comparison despite the fact that CT often preceded MR.

In addition, it is referred to a double blind study of 380 CT and MR brain examinations from the University of Utrecht and Cologne. The results of statistical analysis were presented elsewhere (1).

Emphasis has been put on tumorous and ischemic brain lesions, whereas inflammatory, degenerative or other diseases have been studied less frequently.

RESULTS

I. Detection of Pathology

In our own patients, MRI detected abnormalities in 98% as compared to 88% in CT. The cooperative study revealed a sensitivity of 90% for MR and of 87% for CT. Averaged from both studies, the difference betweeen both procedures was in the range of 8%.

In tumors MRI was superior especially in low grade gliomas, in acoustic neurinomas (Fig.1), in malignant lymphomas (Fig.2), in epidermoids, in arteriovenous malformations and — independent of the histologic diagnosis — in very small lesions. Initial difficulties in detecting extraaxial lesions, especially meningiomas, have been overcome by the use of paramagnetic contrast agents.

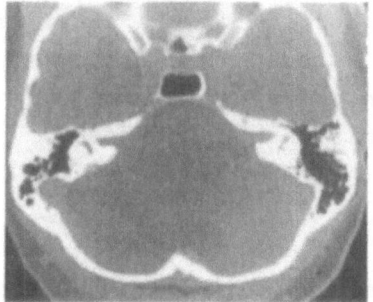 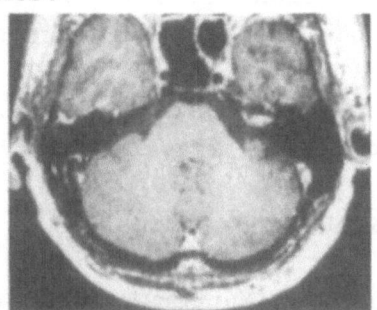

Fig.1: Right intracanalicular acoustic neuroma. a) high resolution CT.b) T1-weigthed SE after Gd-DTPA injection. Extension of tumor can be seen clearly on MRI. By the CT scan one can only speculate about the presence of a tumor, regarding the enlargement of the internal auditory canal.

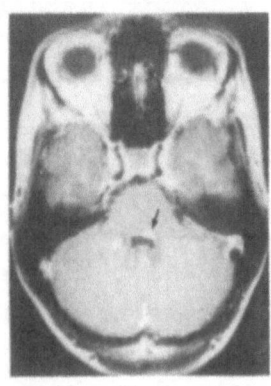

Fig.2: A 24-y-old woman with known malignant lymphoma presented with increasing paresis of the abducens nerve. Contrast-enhanced CT could not explain the complaints. MRI demonstrated involvement of the nucleus n. abducentis (arrow) by the lymphoma (T1-weighted SE after Gd-DTPA injection).

It is well known that demonstration of brain infarcts by CT depends on the stage of infarct. Especially in the acute phase up to 48 hours and around the 14th day ("fogging effect"), ischemic lesions may not be detected by CT. This was not true with MRI in several cases. In addition, MRI proved an extreme high sensitivity for glial scars in the white brain matter of patients with cerebro-vascular disease. These white matter lesions do not correlate with the extent of vascular stenoses or occlusions, shown by angiography.

Beside brain tumors and infarcts there are more diseases, where higher sensitivity of MR helps for efficient diagnosis:

Inflammatory lesions were demonstrated earlier by MR than by CT. This proved especially useful in Herpes encephalitis, which needs specific therapy as soon as possible. In patients with AIDS MR offered advantages for detection even of small lesions due to opportunistic infections like toxoplasmosis (2). However, in several cases of viral meningoencephalitis neither MRI nor CT showed perceptible disease.

Thrombosis of the sagittal sinus, which is hard to recognize by CT, can be diagnosed prima vista by MR.

Subtle subacute and chronic parenchymal hemorrhage and extraaxial hematomas were demonstrated better by MR (Fig.3). On the other hand, acute bleeding is sufficiently diagnosed by CT. Especially patients with acute trauma are much better evaluated in a few seconds by CT than in a few minutes by MR; moreover, in the CT scanner vital functions can be supervised easier.

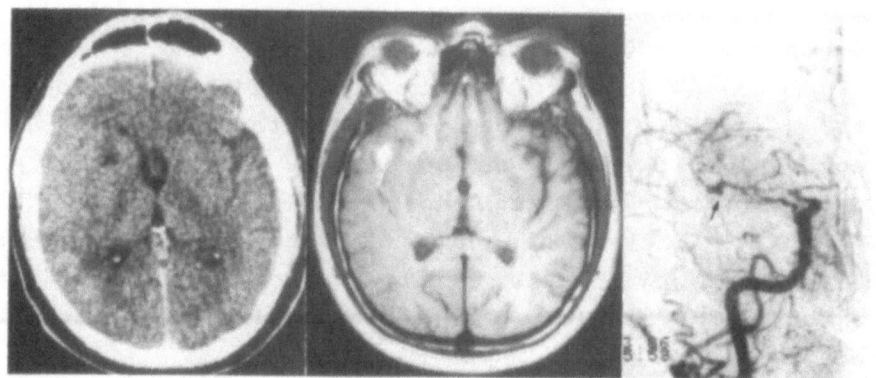

Fig.3: In a 59-y-old man with appropriate clinical signs, MRI clearly demonstrated intraparenchymal and subarachnoid hemorrhage, which was not appreciated on CT 20 hours before. Angiography revealed an aneurysm (arrow) of the Arteria cerebri media.

II. Localization and Delineation of Pathology

The exact determination of tumor extension is very important for planning an operation. The higher soft tissue contrast and the possibility of direct multiplanar imaging is a major advantage of MRI. These features proved even more useful for defining tumor extension than for tumor detection. 28% of all tumors could be localized more precise by MR than by CT.

MR preceded CT especially in intrameatal acoustic neurinomas (compare Fig.1) and in midline and posterior fossa tumors. Differentiation between tumor and perifocal edema was difficult with both imaging modalities. In 36% of our patients peritumorous edema was found. The tumor margin could be differentiated from surrounding edema in 60% by MR and in 62% by CT. The better result of CT results from the more frequent use of contrast agents. In infiltratively growing gliomas (astrocytomas and grade III oligodendrogliomas) it was never possible to delineate an edema even after administration of contrast agents.

In infarcts, necrotic areas could be assigned clearly to the white or grey brain matter. Thus, cortical infarcts could be distinguished from subcortical ones. In the follow-up of infarcts, CT and MR showed similar results.

III. Nature of Lesion

Finally, the specifity of diagnosis was evaluated. Though MRI and CT are based on fundamentally different physical phenomena, information about the length of history, the age and sex of the patient and the neurologic deficits are considered for evaluation beside the form, extension and localization of the lesion. Neither the quantitative evaluation of the signal intensity nor the direct measurements of relaxation times play an important part for establishing the final diagnosis. The reasons for that are the variability of signal intensity and an obvious overlap for different pathologies.

The difficulties of differential diagnosis may be illustrated by the following case:

A 40-year-old man presented with a four month history of partial seizures. CT was normal. MRI showed a small area of increased signal intensity (prolonged T2) without mass effect within the left temporal lobe (Fig. 4).

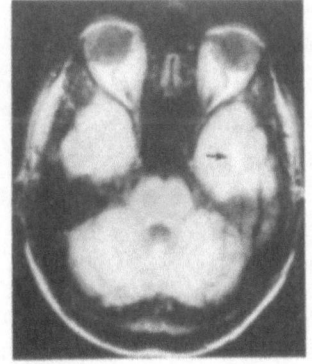

This finding confronts us with problems of differential diagnosis. In 1984, BRADLEY et al. (3) already pointed out the difficulty in differentiating small gliomas and glial scars.

54

Moreover, white matter changes due to traumatic, infectious, or ischemic events have to be considered. The radiologist can establish the diagnosis of a focal brain lesion by MRI, but cannot give a definite advice to the neurosurgeon about the need for an operation.
In the presented case, anticonvulsive therapy failed to control the seizures. Therefore, a surgical resection of the lesion was performed and a glioblastoma found histologically.

There are only few pathologies, which can be characterized definitely by MRI. For example, these are lipomas and flow-related effects. On the other hand, CT proved to be superior for detection of small calcifications (Fig. 5). This may be of special diagnostic value in oligodendrogliomas, meningiomas and other calcified tumors.

Fig.5: Left temporal oligodendroglioma.
CT scan demonstrates small calcifications, which point to the diagnosis. MRI shows extent of the lesion, but reveals an unspecific finding.

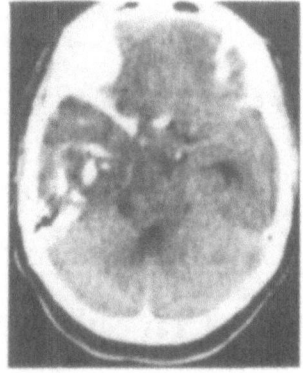 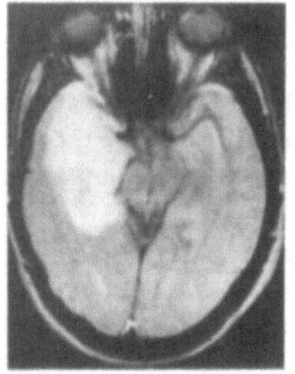

Contrast enhancement — patchy, homogenous or ring-shaped showed similar results in MRI and CT (4), whereby paramagnetic chelates (e.g. Gadolinium—DTPA) are used in MR. We observed only two cases of enhancement, which had not been detected by CT. Corresponding to the experiences of BRANT-

ZAWADZKI et al.(5,6), we did not observe increased sensitivity in intraaxial lesions, but small extraaxial lesions may
be missed without the use of contrast agents.

CONCLUSIONS

1. To our assessment, MRI will be generally accepted in the
primary diagnosis of intracranial pathologies because of its
higher sensitivity. This is especially true for suspected
brain stem lesions and acoustic neurinomas. On the other
hand, one major use of MRI may be the exclusion of perceptible brain disease.

2. With increasing experience in evaluating MR examinations,
an additional CT will not be necessary in most cases. Positive CT will save additional MR vice versa. Therefore, double examinations can be avoided. Only for definite planning
of either surgery or radiation, multidimensional MRI of a
pathologic lesion may be justified. A supplementary MRI for
classification of a lesion seems not to justified, because
the expected results are not better in most cases as compared to CT.

3. For detection of non-tumorous brain lesions MRI is
superior to CT as well. Compared to the suspicion on an intracranial tumor, however, the indication for MRI is less
clear, because characteristic clinical findings (e.g. CSF
changes in encephalitis) often lead to the diagnosis. The
imaging modalities are useful for comfirming the diagnosis,
for localization of the pathologic changes and for exclusion of complications like hemorrhage. In most cases CT can
provide these informations, MRI seems not to be necessary
then.

4. If an intracranial pathology has been recognized and localized, follow-up studies can be performed by CT. Only in rare cases, where MRI was the only imaging modality to show positive findings, this modality should be chosen for control. It is still unclear whether MRI gives better results in the diagnosis of relapse after surgery or radiotherapy. Up to now, our own experiences argue against that.

5. Has MR been used as the primary modality and shall additional CT be avoided, applications of contrast agents in MR gain increasing significance to specify the diagnosis of brain tumors. The role of contrast agents in non-tumorous brain lesions remains to be defined.

6. In traumatology, CT remains the modality of choice, as hemorrhage and bony destruction can be proved or excluded easily and quickly.

ACKNOWLEDGEMENT

This work was supported by the Deutsche Forschungsgemeinschaft (DFG)

REFERENCES

(1) STEINBRICH W, HUYNEN CHJN., den BOER JA, BALERIAUX D, GOODENOUGH DJ, MÖDDER U, MOREIRA PEREIRA RA-
MOS L: Rigorous observer performance evaluation by double blind reading of MR and CT brain studies.
   Society of Magnetic Resonance, 5th Ann Meeting - Montreal 1986, Book of Abstracts 737-738.

(2) KRESTIN GP, JÜRGENS R, STEINBRICH W, DIEDERICH N: Zerebrale Beteiligung bei erworbenem Immunman-
gelsyndrom (AIDS) - Computertomographie (CT) und Kernspintomographie (MR).
   Fortschr. Röntgenstr. (1986) 145: 625-630.

(3) BRADLEY WG, WALUCH V, YADLEY R, WYCOFF RR: Comparison of CT and MR in 400 Patients with Suspected
Disease of the Brain and Cervical Spinal Cord.
   Radiology (1984) 152: 695-702.

(4) HEINDEL W, STEINBRICH W, FRIEDMANN G: Magnetische Resonanztomographie (MR) bei Hirntumoren - Ge-
genüberstellung der Ergebnisse Multiechotechnik und Gadolinium-DPTA.
   Fortschr. Röntgenstr. (1986) 145: 158-162.

(5) BRANT-ZAWADZKI M, BERRY I, OSAKI L, BRASCH R, MUROVIC J, NORMAN D: Gd-DTPA in Clinical MR of the
Brain: 1. Intraaxial Lesions.
   AJR (1986) 147: 1223-1230.

(6) BERRY I, BRANT-ZAWADZKI M, OSAKI L, BRASCH R, MUROVIC J, NEWTON TH: Gd-DTPA in Clinical MR of the
Brain: 2. Extraaxial Lesions and Normal Structures.
   AJR (1986) 147: 1231-1235.

PET AND MR IMAGING OF THE BRAIN

ROBERT M. KESSLER

INTRODUCTION

Both MRI and PET are computer-assisted cross-sectional imaging modalities which do not utilize transmitted x-rays. MRI studies of the brain to date have largely used proton studies for imaging. These studies image mobile protons and the images created are dependent on T1 and T2 relaxation times, spin density, and, to an extent, bulk flow. In the brain, much of the contrast seen on proton MRI is due to brain water content and the state of water molecules (1). The images obtained with proton MRI have given clinical information regarding the anatomy of the brain, pathological changes, and limited information regarding chemical composition and flow. PET utilizes physiologically active radiopharmaceuticals labelled with positron-emitting isotopes (11C, 13N, 15O, 18F) to study metabolic functions in man. Positron emission tomography provides quantitative cross-sectional images of radioisotope distribution. Tracer kinetic models are used to convert measurements of isotope concentration into measures of metabolic function such as glucose metabolic rate, cerebral blood flow or protein synthesis in normal and abnormal tissue.

MRI has been widely utilized for clinical diagnosis of central nervous system disease. PET has been widely utilized in brain research but has been utilized less extensively for clinical diagnosis. PET has been shown to have clinical utility in the diagnosis of gliomas, epilepsy, stroke and dementia. An examination of the contributions of each modality in these disorders illustrate the role of each in clinical diagnosis.

Gliomas

MRI has been shown to have high sensitivity in detecting cerebral neoplasms. Gliomas typically have elongated T1's, T2's and usually enhance following IV administration of GdDTPA. The enhancement of gliomas with GdDTPA has been shown to be greater in high grade gliomas than in low grade tumors (2). One of the difficulties with both CT and MRI studies of gliomas has been the difficulty of separating tumor and the surrounding zones of tumor infiltration from edema (3) and in distinguishing post-radiation changes from tumor recurrence (4,5).

PET has utilized 18F labelled 2 fluorodeoxyglucose (18FDG) to study glycolysis and 11C labelled methionine to study protein synthesis in cerebral gliomas. 18FDG studies have shown that, relative to normal grey matter, high grade gliomas have higher 18FDG uptake and low grade gliomas have relatively lower uptake (6). 18FDG studies have proved useful in distinguishing recurrent tumor from radiation necrosis (7); radiation necrosis has decreased 18FDG uptake while recurrent high grade tumors have increased uptake. 11c-amino acids studies have shown increased uptake in tumors and in the infiltrating zone of tumors compared to areas of edema (8,9). MRI studies have not been capable of distinguishing these (4).

The studies performed to date would suggest that MRI is the initial

study of choice for detection of cerebral gliomas. If biopsy is con-
templated, 18FDG studies can help to direct the biopsy to the area of the
neoplasm of greatest malignancy. 11C animo acid studies may be useful for
determining extent of tumor for surgical resection or radiation therapy.
For follow-up studies, MRI and PET are needed for complete evaluation.

Epilepsy

Partial seizures, which in many cases can progress to generalized seizures, are often caused by focal abnormalities in the brain. MRI has been
used in several studies to detect structural abnormalities in patients
with seizures. These structural abnormalities include tumors, vascular
malformations, medial temporal sclerosis, hamartomas, and posttraumatic
scarring (10). In cases of partial seizures, about 40% of cerebral MRI
studies reveal some abnormality (11,12,13). As has been indicated by a
recent case presented by Theodore (13), abnormalities on MRI need to be
correlated with EEG findings as the presence of an abnormality does not
establish it to be the cause of seizures.

PET studies with 18FDG have consistently identified foci of decreased
glucose metabolism interictally which correspond to the seizure focus in
from 50 to 75% of patients (13,14). During seizure activity, increased
glucose metabolism has been seen at the seizure focus. Decreased interictal glucose metabolism can be caused by a number of insults to the brain,
and so correlating EEG findings, both maximal interictal spikes and locus
of ictal onset activity, are need to confirm a hypometabolic focus as
being epileptogenic.

In partial seizures, the initial imaging study should be a MRI: if this
proves negative or equivocal, then a 18 FDG PET study should be performed.
Both of these studies need to be correlated with EEG studies.

Dementia

In the United States, the fraction of the population over age 60 is
steadily increasing and the prevalence of dementia in the general population is rising. At present, some 600,000 persons in the United States are
severely demented while an additional 1.4 million have a mild or moderate
dementia (15). In 50-60% of cases of dementia the cause is Alzheimer's
Disease. The remainder of dementia cases are due to multinfarct dementia
by itself and with Alzheimer's Disease, alcoholic dementia, Huntington's
disease, subcortical arteriosclerotic encephalopathy, depression, drug
intoxication and a variety of other causes. The most frequent differential
diagnosis is between Alzheimer's Disease, vascular related dementia and
treatable causes of dementia such as depression or drug intoxication.

MRI can provide important information for the diagnosis of multi-infarct
dementia, subcortical arteriosclerotic encephalopathy, and Hungtinton's
disease. MRI findings in Alzheimer's Disease are nondiagnostic; often some
cortical atrophy, ventricular enlargement and some white matter disease is
seen (16). In 60% of Alzheimers's patients, there is pathological evidence
of white matter disease which is similar to subcortical arteriosclerotic
encephalopathy which will be discussed below (17). PET with 18FDG
(18,19,20), H2150 and 1502 (21) has shown reduced cerebral metabolism
particularly in the parietal and temporal lobes, usually bilaterally: the

lobes have similarly reduced metabolism in some cases. The primary soma-
tosensory cortex, basal ganglia and thalamus are relatively spared. The
presence of these characteristic metabolic deficits on PET studies combined with athrophy and mild to moderate ventricular enlargement on MRI
strongly suggest the diagnosis of Alzheimer's Disease.

MRI has proved efficacious in the diagnosis of white matter disease. The
frequent findings of white matter abnormalities in elderly individuals
(22) has led to a heightened awareness of subcortical arteriosclerotic
encephalopathy (SAE) (23,24,25,26). Pathologically characterized by demyelination, a loss of axons and glial cells, and a hyaline arterio-
losclerosis of the small perforating arteries of the white matter, it is
seen on MRI as areas on increased signal on T2 weighted pulse sequences in
the periventricular white matter and in the centrum semiovale. These
changes are more frequently but not invariably seen in subjects with hypertension and/or atherosclerotic vascular disease. Clinically patients
with SAE can present with dementia, motor disturbances including gait abnormalities and pseudobulbar palsy, incontinence, psychological disturbances, strokes, and focal neurological disturbances which can evolve
acutely or subacutely (25,26). MRI is the diagnostic modality of choice in
this entity. Similar changes, both pathological (17) and on MRI (16) have
been reported in Alzheimer's subjects. PET studies in SAE have not been
reported.

Cerebrovascular Disease

Stroke is an extremely common disorder. Both PET and MRI studies of
stroke can provide diagnostic information. MRI studies have shown regions
of prolonged T1 and T2 in stroke as early as 6 hours after the clinical
event (27,28). These findings are presumably due to the rapid onset of
cytotoxic edema. With subsequent vasogenic edema starting within the first
day, the area of abnormal signal increases and edema spreads into the
white matter (29). As the vasogenic edema progresses, the area of abnormal
signal and mass effect reach a maximum by day three to four days and then
regress. A residual region of increased T1 and T2 is generally seen.

With PET, studies of cerebral blood flow (CBF) and oxygen metabolism
have shown an orderly progression of findings (30,31,32). With a fall in
CBF, there is an initial vasodilatation and a slowing of the cerebral
vascular transit time. With further falls in CBF, the oxygen extraction
fraction rises. If CBF falls to levels less than 15ml/100 grams/min,
energy failure occurs (33) and with it the rapid onset of cytotoxic edema
occurs. Cerebral tissue remains viable for many minutes after the onset of
energy failure. In some animal studies viability of many cells has remai-
ned for up to an hour (34,35). The role of PET in the diagnosis of most
cases of acute cerebrovascular disease is not critical because of the lack
of therapy. PET has a role in the evaluation of patients for extra cra-
nial-intracranial bypass studies, particularly those patients with
orthostatic symptoms. It will probably be of use in the evaluation of patients with vasculitis for monitoring therapy and in the evaluation cerebrovascular spasm after subarachnoid hemorrhage. If a therapy can be
found to minimize the spread of infarction into the ischemic penumbra
surrounding an area of infarction, then PET would be important for the
monitoring of this therapy.

Summary

   PET and proton MRI imaging provide different types of diagnostic information. MRI gives exquisite anatomic information, information regarding
tissue water composition, and limited information about chemical composition. PET can provide physiological data regarding regional energy metabolism, protein synthesis, and cerebral neurotransmission. These modalities are more often complimentary than competitive. MRI studies of sodium,
lactate and phosphorus may provide information regarding tissue energy
metabolism that is more directly competitive with PET. PET howver can
study physiological processes which occur at extremely low concentrations,
e.g., neurotransmitter function, protein synthesis, and it is unlikely
that MRI will be competitive in these studies. For the immediate future
PET and MRI provide complimentary information regarding disease states.

REFERENCES

1. Kato H, Kogure K, Ohotomo et al: Characterization of experimental
    ischemic brain edema using proton nuclear magnetic resonance imaging.
    J Cereb Blood Flow Metabolism 6:212-221, 1986.

2. Graif M, Bydder GM, Steiner RE et al: Contrast enhanced MR imaging of
    malignant brain tumors. AJNR 6:855-862, 1985.

3. Burger PC: Pathologic anatomy and CT correlations in glioblastoma
    multiforme. Appl Neurophysiol 46:180-187, 1983.

4. Domms GC, Hecht S. Brandt-Zawdzki M et al: Brain radiation lesions: MR
    imaging. Radiology 158:149-155, 1986.

5. Brismar J, Roberson GH, Davis KR: Radiation necrosis of the brain.
    Neuroradiology 12:109-113, 1976.

6. Di Chiro G, De La Paz RL, Brooks RA et al: Glucose utilization of ce-
    rebral gliomas measured by [18F] fluorodeoxyglucose and positron
    emission tomography. Neurology 32:1323-1329, 1982.

7. Patronas NJ, Di Chiro G, Brooks RA et al:Work in progress: [18F]
    fluorodeoxyglucose and positron emission tomography in the evaluation
    of radiation necrosis of the brain. Radiology 144:885-889, 1982.

8. Ericson K, Lilja A, Bergstron M et al: Positron emission tomography
    with ([/C] methl) -L-methionine (11C) D-glucose and [68GaEDTA] in
    supratentorial tumors. J Comp Asst Tomogr 9:683-689, 1985.

9. Lilja A, Bergstrom K, Hartvig P et al: Dynamic study of supratentorial
    gliomas with L-methyl-11C-methionine and positron emission tomography.
    AJNR 6:505-514, 1985.

10. Adams RD, Victor M: Epilepsy and other convulsive states, in Princip-
    les of Neurology, Second edition, pp. 211-230, McGraw Hill, New York,
    1981.

11. Lessor RP, Modic MT, Weinstein MA et al: Magnetic resonance imaging
    (1.5 Tesla) in patients with intractable focal seizures. Arch Neurol
    43:367-371, 1986.

12. Jabbari B, Gunderson CH, Wippold F et al: Magnetic resonance imaging in partial complex epilepsy. Arch Neurol 43:869-872, 1986.

13. Theodore WH, Dorwart R, Holmes M et al: Neuroimaging in refractory partial seizure: comparison of PET, CT, and MRI. Neurology 36:750-759.

14. Engel J Jr, Kuhl DE, Phelps ME et al: Comparative localization of epileptic foci in partial epilepsy by PCT and EEG. Ann Neurol 12:529-537, 1982.

15. Katzman R: Alzheimer's Disease. New England J Med 314:964-973, 1986.

16. George AE, deLeon MJ, Kalnin A et al: Leukoencephalopathy in normal and pathologic aging: 2. MRI of brain lucencies. AJR 7:567-570, 1986.

17. Brun A, Englund E: A white matter disorder in dementia of the Alzheimer type: a pathoanatomical study. Ann Neurol 19:253-262, 1986.

18. Foster NL, Chase TN, Fedio P et al: Alzheimer's Disease: focal cortical changes shown by positron emission tomography. Neurology (NY) 33:9651-9665, 1983.

19. Friedland RP, Budinger TF, Gary E et al: Regional cerebral metabolic alterations in dementia of the Alzheimer type: positron tomography with [18F] fluorodeoxyglucose. J Comp Assist Tomogr 7:590-598, 1983.

20. Benson DF, Kuhl DE, Hawkins RA et al: The FDG scan in Alzheimer and multi-infarct dementia. Arch Neurol 40:711-713, 1983.

21. Frakowiak RJS, Pozilli C, Legg NJ et al: Regional cerebral oxygen supply and utilization in dementia-clinical and physiological study with oxygen-15 and positron tomography. Brain 104:753-778, 1980.

22. Bradley WG, Waluch V, Brant-Zawadzki M et al: Patchy periventricular white matter lesions in the elderly: common observation during NMR imaging. Noninvasive Med Imaging 1:35-41, 1984.

23. Kinkel WR, Jacobs L, Ploachini H et al: Subcortical arteriosclerotic encephalopathy (Binswanger's disease), computed tomographic nuclear magnetic resonance, and clinical correlations. Arch Neurol 42:951-959, 1985.

24. Brant-Zawadzki M, Fein G, Van Dyke C et al: MR imaging of the aging brain: patchy white matter lesions and dementia. AJNR 6:675-682, 1985.

25. Caplan LR, Schoene WC: Clinical features of subcortical arteriosclerotic encephalopathy (Binswanger's disease). Neurology 28:1206-1215, 1978.

26. Loizou LA, Kendall BE, Marshall J: Subcortical arteriosclerotic encephalopathy: a clinical and radiological investigation. J Neurology Neurosurgery and Psychiatry 44:294-304, 1981.

27. Sipponen JT, Kaste M, Ketoneu L et al: Serial nuclear magnetic resonance (NMR) imaging in patients with cerebral infarction. J Comput Assist Tomogr 7:585-589, 1983.

28. Bryan RN, Willcott MR, Schneiders NJ et al: Nuclear magnetic resonance, evaluation of stroke. Radiology 149:189-192, 1983.

29. Hossman KA: Experimental aspects of stroke in vascular disease of the central nervous system, ed. by RWR Russell, Churchill Livingstone, New York, 1983, p.73-100.

30. Lenzi GL, Frakowiak RJS, Jones T: Cerebral oxygen metabolism and blood flow in human cerebral ischemic infarction: J Comp Assist Tomogr 2:321-333, 1982.

31. Wise RJS, Bernardi S, Frakowiak RJS et al: Serial observations on the pathophysiology of acute stroke. Brain 106:197-222, 1983.

32. Gibbs JM, Wise RJ, Leenders KL, Jones T: Evaluation of cerebral perfusion reserve in patients with carotid artery occlusion. Lancet 1:310-314, 1984.

33. Powers WJ, Grubb RL, Darriet D, Raichle ME: Cerebral blood flow and cerebral metabolic rate of oxygen requirements for cerebral function and viability in humans. J Cereb Blood Flow Metabolism 5:600-608, 1985.

34. Hossman KA, Ophoff BG: Recovery of monkey brain after prolonged ischemia. I Electrophysiology and Brain Electrolytes. J Cereb Blood Flow Metabolism 6:15-21, 1986.

35. Bodsch W, Barbier A, Oehmichen M, Ophoff BG, Hossman KA: Recovery of monkey brain after prolonged ischemia. II Protein synthesis and morphological alterations. J Cereb Blood Flow Metabolism 6:23-33, 1986.

COMPARATIVE STUDY OF MRI VERSUS CT FOR THE DIAGNOSTIC WORK UP OF LESIONS
IN THE NOSE AND PARANASAL SINUSES.

R.G.M. DE SLEGTE (1), G.J. GERRITSEN (2), J.J. NAUTA (3), M.B. HOEN (1),
F.C. CREZEE (1),

Free University Hospital, Amsterdam
(1) Department of Neuroradiology and Radiology
(2) Department of medical statistics
(3) Department of Otolaryngology & Head and Neck Surgery

ABSTRACT
Staging of malignant tumours of the nasal cavity and paranasal sinuses
was studied in a total of 36 patients using Computed Tomography (CT) and
Magnetic Resonance Imaging (MRI). Areas affected by the tumour were
studied and clinical staging was carried out using CT and MRI
separately. For most cases, surgical findings were also available and
could be used for comparison. In a number of cases (n=13) in which the
lesions were due to benign lesions, the results of MRI and CT were also
compared with one another and if possible with surgical findings. The
results of CT and MRI were compared by statistical analysis.

INTRODUCTION
Malignancies of the nose and paranasal sinuses constitute some 0.2-0.3%
of all tumours and 3% of all head and neck tumours. The most frequently
occurring malignancies are squamous cell-, adenoidcystic- and
adenocarcinomas; these epithelial malignancies are known for their
invasive growth (4, 8). The diagnostic work-up of these tumours requires
a thorough assessment of their location and extension into adjacent
areas in order to plan appropriate treatment.
In attempts to perform diagnosis non-invasively, it has long been the
practice to perform plain radiography and polytomography to define the
extent of the tumour. Computed Tomography (CT) has proven to be a
diagnostic tool in the diagnosis of lesions of the nasal cavity and
paranasal sinuses (3, 4, 7, 8, 13). Magnetic Resonance Imaging(MRI) has
been shown to possess advantages over other imaging methods in a variety
of anatomical regions including the central nervous system and the

musculoskeletal system.In this retrospective study, an attempt has been made to evaluate and compare CT and MRI results as a pre-operative diagnostic tool. A blind study has been performed on 36 E.N.T.-patients with (suspected) lesions of the paranasal sinuses or nasal cavity. Evaluation of CT and MRI examinations of the lesions and assessment of tumour extension into 5 different compartments was performed. The results of MRI and CT scan examinations were compared to the surgical findings and the results of histopathological studies of the resected specimen. A statistical analysis of the results was carried out.

METHODS AND METERIAL

During the period 1985-1986 thirty-six patients with suspected or proven lesions of the paranasal sinuses, nose or facial bones (excluding primary tumours of the orbita). They were examined with preferably both CT scanning and MR imaging to evaluate the extend of the lesions. There were 20 males and 16 females, their ages varying from 18-90 years. Histopathological staging of specimens established that 23 lesions were malignant and 13 were non-malignant (table 1). These malignant cases consisted of 6 squamous cell carcinoma, 6 adenoid cystic carcinoma, 2 adenocarcinoma, 3 rhabdomyosarcoma, 1 fibrosarcoma, 3 melanoma, 1 chondrosarcoma and 1 fibrous histiocytoma.

Thirty-one of the 36 patients underwent both investigative methods, followed by surgical resection in 27 cases. Four patients received no surgical treatment because of extensive tumour-growth through the skull-base or, as in the case of a rhabdomyosarcoma, because the primary choice of therapy was chemotherapy .

Three of the 36 patients underwent one of the two investigative methods plus surgical resection. On MRI, one case showed no obvious tumour mass but a sinusitis. The patient refused further CT examination. In one case, MRI failed because the patient suffered from claustrophobia which made examination impossible. Another case did not undergo MRI as conventional X-rays and CT-scan confirmed osteoma of the frontal sinus. Hence, 6 cases were excluded from the comparative study as they did not fulfill all criteria for inclusion.

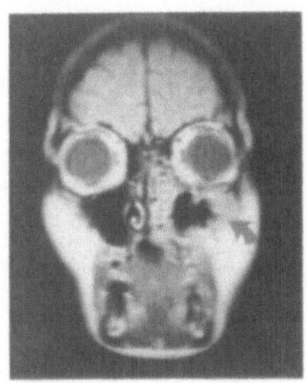

FIGURE 1A

Example of extension into the soft tissues of the cheek in a 45 year old woman with an adenoidcystic carcinoma.
Coronal MRI 1 cm slice-thickness. TR 1500 TE32 2nd echo. Tumor involvement of the laterocaudal wall of the maxillary sinus and upper jaw (arrow).

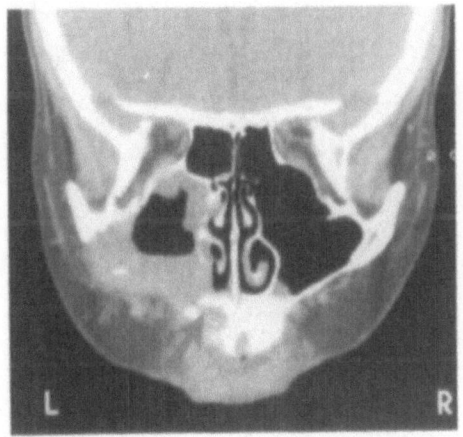

FIGURE 1B

Direct coronal CT section (3mm slice-thickness) obvious tumor involvement of the soft tissues of the cheek (small arrow) and upper jaw (big arrow).

68

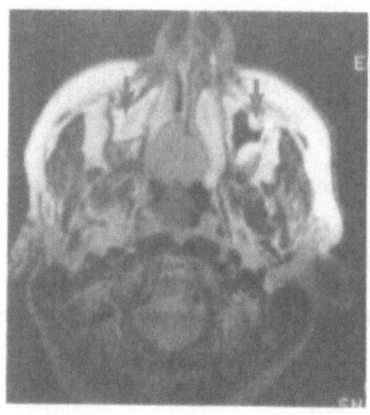

FIGURE 2A

Giant cell tumor of the palatum in a girl with a hyperparathyrodia due
to adenoma. Axial MRI section 0.4 cm slice-thickness TR 1500, - TE90,
2 nd echo. Good delineation of the tumor (arrow head) with mucosal
swelling of the maxillary sinuses (arrow).

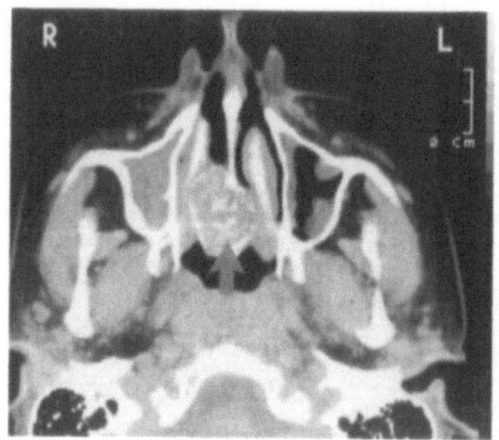

FIGURE 2B

Axial CT scan 3mm slice thickness good visualization of the tumor
(arrow), with bone structures in the tumor which leads to diagnosis of a
bony tumor. Giant cell tumor (not possible with MRI).

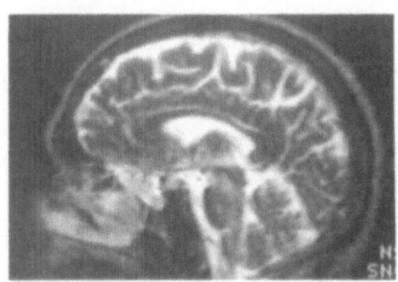

FIGURE 3A

A 61 year old woman with involvement of anterior ethmoidal cells by
tumor (location 3).

Sagittal MRI section. 1 cm slice-thickness TR 2000, TE 256, 8th of 8
echos. The tumor can be diagnosed (arrow head) and be seperated of the
mucosal swelling (arrow).

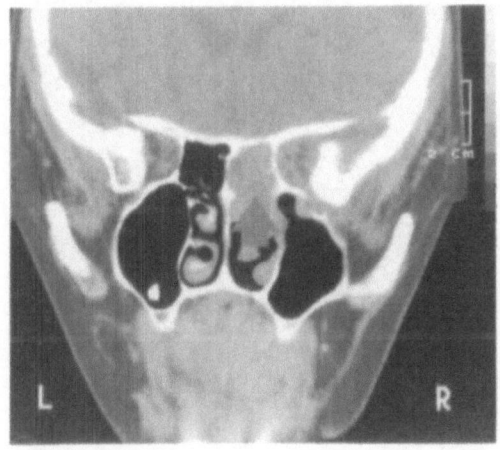

FIGURE 3B

Direct coronal CT scan 3 mm slice-thickness; destruction of the floor of
the anterior ethmoid cells (arrow head); soft tissue differentation
between tumor and mucosal swelling is not possible.

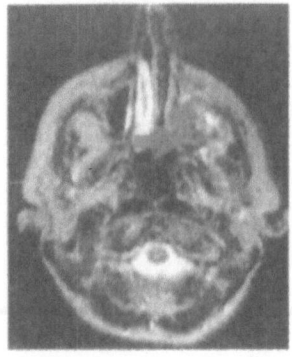

FIGURE 4A

42 year old woman with a malignant fibrocytic histioma, which had
developed 41 years after previous radiotherapy for retinoblastoma of the
eye. Tumor extension into the infratemporal fossa.

Axial MRI section 1 cm slice thickness. The tumor has a low signal
intensity area (big arrow), the normal anatomy of the infratemporal
fossa is distorted (small arrow).

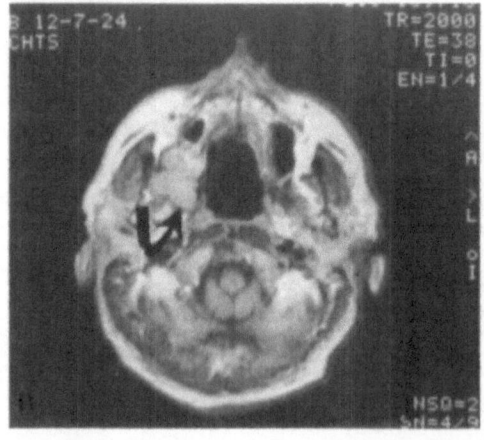

FIGURE 4B

For comparison: a 5 mm thick section of an angioma of the upper jaw with
a more T1 weighted image. Due to the 5mm slice-thickness a better
spatial resolution and thus better visualization of the infratemporal
fossa is obtained (arrow).

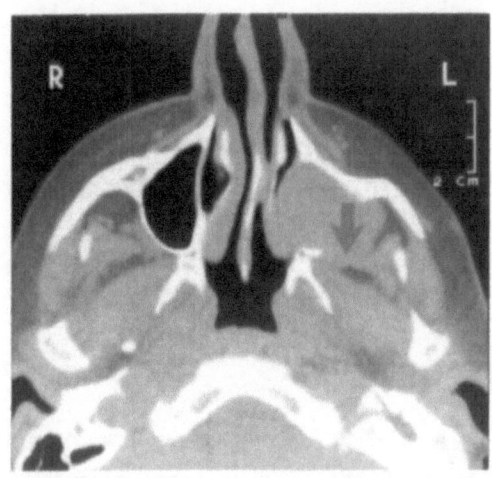

FIGURE 4C

High resolution section in the same patient as 4. Obvious involvement of the infratemporal fossa (arrows).

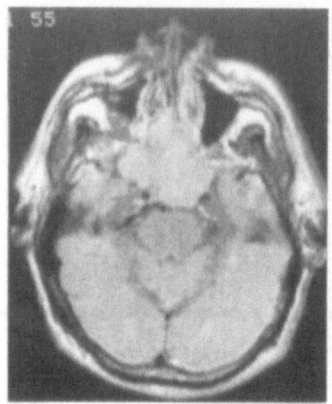

FIGURE 5A

A 64 year old man with tumour involvement of the clivus, parasellar
region by squamouscellcarcinoma (location 5).
Axial MRI section 1 cm slice-thickness TR1500, TE60, 1st of two echo's.
Tumourinvolvement of infratemporal fossa, clivus and para sellar region
(arrows)

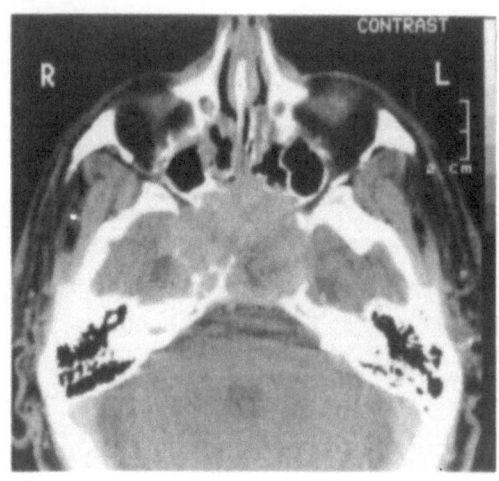

FIGURE 5B
CT scan on the same level for comparison.

TABLE 1: Distribution of pathology in 36 cases

Malignant		non-malignant	
diagnosis	frequency n=23	diagnosis	frequency n=13
squamous cell	6 (26.1%)	sinusitis	3
adenocystic	6 (26.1%)	heamangioma	2
rhabdomyosarcoma	3 (13%)	papilloma inversum	2
melanoma	3 (13%)	osteoma	1
adenocarcinoma	2 (8.7%)	ameloblastoma	1
fibrosarcoma	1 (4.3%)	encephalocèle	1
chondrosarcoma	1 (4.3%)	choanal polyps	1
radio-induced	1 (4.3%)	giant cell tumour	1
fibrous histiocytoma		no lesion at all	1

Methods

The CT examinations were performed on a Philips 350 Tomoscan (high
resolution mode). The slices were taken in 2 directions: transverse and
direct coronal with a slice thickness of 3 mm and a slice-increment of 6
mm. If necessary 3 mm consecutive slices were made.
The MR Images were made on a 0.6 tesla Technicare (now General Electric)
superconductive system in transverse, coronal and often in sagittal
directions. A varied range of pulse sequences was used, the most
frequent being:
- Inversion Recovery/Spin Echo (IR):
  TI 400, TR 1400, TE 30 msec (multiple slices)
- Saturation Recovery/Spin Echo (SE):
  TR 500, TE 30 and 60 msec (2 echos)(multiple slices)
  TR 1500, TE 30 and 60 msec (2 echos)(multiple slices)
  TR 2000, TE 30 to 240 msec (1-8 echos)(single slices)

Staging

Tumours considered to arise within the maxillary sinus were staged
according to the American Joint Committee classification system (12).
The tumours that originated at the alveolar ridge or upper jaw were
staged as maxillary sinus tumours.
In this classification T1 tumours are confined to the mucosa of the
infrastructure; T2 tumours are confined to the mucosa of the

suprastructure or produce medial or inferior bony wall destruction; T3 tumours invade the skin, orbit, anterior ethmoid sinus or pterygoid muscle and T4 tumours extend to the cribiforme plate, posterior ethmoids, sphenoids, nasopharynx, pterygoid plate or base of the skull. In tumours of the maxillary sinuses, destruction of more than one maxillary wall is common (5, 8). On admission, most cases will present with a tumour at stage T2 or even a more advanced stage, as was found in our cases.

The most important function of CT or MRI is in demonstrating that the tumour has extended beyond the limits of surgical resection.

Equally important is the demonstration of involvement of vital structures that require more radical surgical approaches such as orbital exenteration (7). Therefore, for practical reasons in this study the area affected by the tumour were divided into 5 locations, which means that T3 tumour was splitted in two stages (stage 3, 4). For the E.N.T. Department of our hospital, extension to location 1, 2 or 3 indicate that radical surgery should be attempted.

The five locations employed were as follows:

1. Involvement of upper jaw or soft tissues of the cheek.
2. Involvement of the medial wall of the maxillary sinus with tumour extension into the nasal cavity or palatum.
3. Involvement of the anterior ethmoidal cells and or orbital wall destruction; or primary tumour localized in ethmoidal or frontal sinuses.
4. Involvement of pterygopalatine fossa, infratemporal fossa or nasopharynx (contra indication for surgery).
5. Involvement of the middle cranial fossa, cribiforme plate, clivus or skull base (contra indication for surgery).

For the 30 patients who underwent CT-scanning and the 29 patients who underwent MR imaging, not all data could be interpreted. The number (n) of patients actually used is given in table 4.

In table 4, the Prevalence and the Predictive Values are given for each location. Unlike the Sensitivity and Specificity, the Predictive Values not only depend on the quality of the test but also on the Prevalence. The Prevalence of extension was lowest for location 5 (through skull base T4) and highest for location 2 (nasal cavity T2).

TABLE 4 Prevalence and Predictive Values

	Prevalence	Method 1 (+/- taken as +)		Method 2 (+/- taken as -)	
		+PV*	-P**	+PV*	-PV**
Location 1					
(n=25)	60%				
CT		100%	91%	100%	83%
MRI		100%	83%	100%	77%
Location 2					
(n=26)	69%				
CT		100%	80%	100%	67%
MRI		94%	70%	93%	58%
Location 3					
(n=25)	48%				
CT		92%	92%	92%	92%
MRI		90%	80%	89%	75%
Location 4					
(n=23)	22%				
CT		63%	100%	67%	94%
MRI		57%	94%	75%	89%
Location 5					
(n=24)	13%				
CT		100%	100%	100%	100%
MRI		100%	95%	100%	95%

* +PV: positive Predictive Value
** -PV: negative Predictive Value

DISCUSSION

Clinical staging has its limitations. The ability of CT to delineate the extent of tumours is well known (3, 4, 5, 7, 8, 9). In this study, the ability of MRI to delineate the extent of a tumour was compared with that of CT and results of histopathological findings.
For practical purposes the extension of a tumour was evaluated for five different locations.
The incidence of tumour extension into the five locations is shown in

76

table 4.
The upper jaw and soft tissues of the cheek (location 1) were involved
in 60% of the cases (Fig. 1).
The region of the upper jaw was best visualized on the coronal views,
however, if dental fillings are present, this can obscure the picture.
The region of the cheek was better visualized on the axial vieuws. If
the dental fillings are paramagnetic, as in one of our cases, the MRI
picture also shows artefacts (Fig. 10). The predictive values of CT and
MRI did not differ significantly for this region.

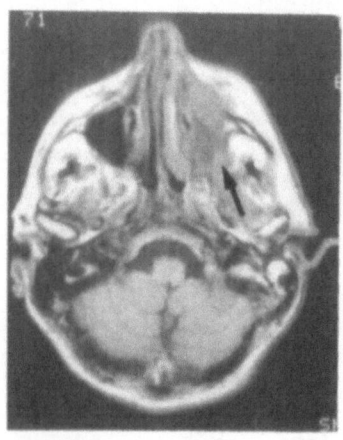

FIGURE 6
T1 weighted image 7.5cm. MRI image demonstrates tumour extension into
the infratemporal fossa. Histopathological examination of the resected
tumour didn't demonstrate tumour extension outside the maxillary sinus.

The nasal cavity and palatum (location 2) were found to be involved in
69% of our cases, the highest percentage found for all locations. If on
CT examination the medial wall of the maxillary sinus was found to be
damaged and a soft tissue mass was present in the maxillary sinus and in
the nasal cavity, the findings were considered to be positive.
If on MRI examination T2 weighted images were made, clear distinction
between tumor and sinusitis was possible (Fig. 2). This is not always
possible in CT scan examinations without the use of intravenous contrast
enhancement. Also for this location no significant differences in
predictive values were found between CT and MRI examination.
In our clinic involvement of the anterior ethmoidal cells and/or orbital

involvement anteriorly located, (location 3) do not form a
contra-indication for curative radical resection; however, an orbital
exentaration has to be performed.

On CT scan examination, destruction of the bony structures of the
anterior ethmoid cells, and/or interruption of the orbital ring on the
caudo-medial side, with or without soft tissue mass extending into the
orbit, were considered as stage 3.

Extension into the ethmoid, however, is difficult to separate from
mucosal swelling and/or sinusitis. The presence of septal bone
destruction was the most important radiological sign on CT examination
(Fig. 3).

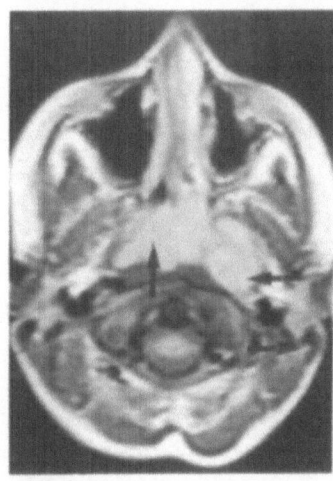

FIGURE 7

Large rhabdomyosarcoma in a 2-year-old child. Tumour extending into the
inferior part of the petrosal bone and contra-lateral side of the
nasopharynx and parapharyngeal space.

On MRI examination, the T2 weighted image can distinguish between tumor
and sinusitis; which is not always possible with CT. The prevalence of
involvement in this area was 48%; there were no significant differences
in the predictive values of CT and MRI.

The prevalence of involvement in location four was 22%. The
infratemporal fossa lies lateral to the parapharyngeal space, is
bordered anteriorly by the maxillary antrum and laterally by the
zygomatic arch and parotid gland. Within the fossa, the medial and
lateral pterygoid muscle, masseter muscle and their envelopping small

78

amounts of fat are symmetrical (in appearance).

On CT scan examination, interruption of the posterior part of the
maxillary antrum, disturbance of normal fat planes, and asymmetric
volume increase of muscle parts was considered to be positive for
involvement (Fig. 4).

On MRI, the various soft tissues of the infratemporal fossa do
contribute to excellent image quality and hence distinction between
normal and pathological anatomy in this region. However,subtle cortical
disruption can not be visualized due to a lack of signal from cortical
bone and difficulty with volume averaging using a section of 7 mm or
more (Fig. 4).

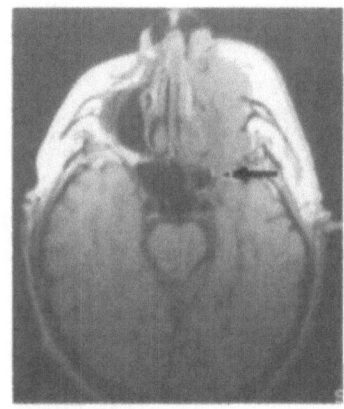

FIGURE 8
Tumour extension in the parasellar region and middle cranial fossa.
Inspite of slice-thickness of 5mm is the extension of the tumour
difficult to see.

The infratemporal fossa was best visualized on the axial vieuws. Obvious
extension of tumour in these region form a contra indication for a
radical surgical approach.At the fourth location, the predictive values
of CT and MRI examination for involvement of the infratemporal fossa and
fossa pterygopalatina and nasopharynx are considerably lower than the
other regions.

The possible explanation is that histopathological staging is difficult
to obtain in tumours of the paranasal sinuses, on surgery tumour
removing is not possible but the tumour will be taken out in particles.

Especially, the posterior part of the maxillary sinus is a difficult area for surgery and histopathological staging. If the histopathological examination of the resected tumour was negative and the results of CT and MRI were positive, the results of CT and MRI were considered as false positive. However, we are not sure that this is a valid interpretation.

Extension through the skull base, the lamina cribosa, clivus, and or parasellar region was present in only 13%, which means that radiotherapy, sometimes in combination with tumor debulking, was the therapy of choice. In our limited experience we found that the parasellar region and interruptions of the middle cranial fossa are less well depicted on the MRI images. CT has the advantage of good visualization of the cancelous bone, with MRI cancelous bone being imaged a low signal (Fig. 8). Moreover only direct extension of a tumour can be visualized.

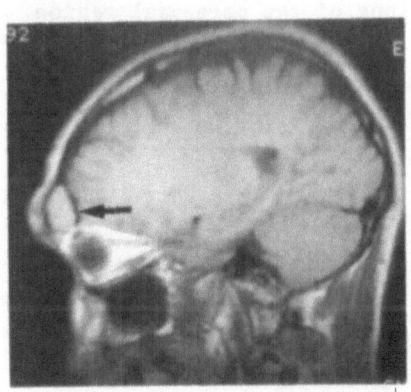 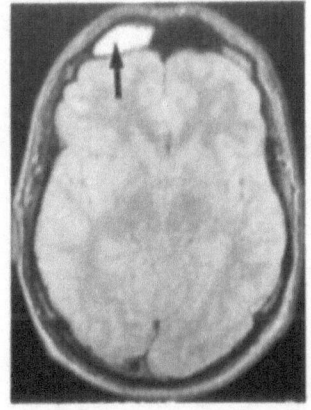

FIGURE 9A+B
A 45 year old man presented with a local bulging above the right eye. MRI demonstrated obvious the nature of this lesion a mucocèle.

Our comparative series is small; there were no differences in the predictive values of CT and MRI.

In conclusion; in this small series, no significant differences were found between these two imaging methods (CT and MRI).

CT has proven to be a good diagnostic mode for E.N.T pathology, however, no spectacular further development is expected in contrast to the

80

situation with MRI.
In general MRI gives the same information about tumour extension as CT.
However, MRI is the diagnostic method that provides some information
about the compounds of lesions (2, 9, 10, 11, 14, 15), T2 weighted
images allow better distinction between tumour and sinusitis. However,
in the present situation MRI is not superior to CT in the evaluation of
destruction of thin bony structures, such as the walls of the antrum,
the cribiforme plate and the lamina papyracea.
Further development of MRI will result in a decrease in the partial
volume effect and in a smaller slice thickness, producing more precise
information about extension of a tumour into different locations.
The use of paramagnetic contrast agents is perhaps less promising in
tumours of the paranasal sinuses, since enhancement of mucosal swelling
seems to obscure the tumour enhancement.
Further evaluation of the comparison between the two imaging modalities
is necessary, but at present no significant differences between CT and
MRI can be demonstrated in staging of lesions of the paranasal region.

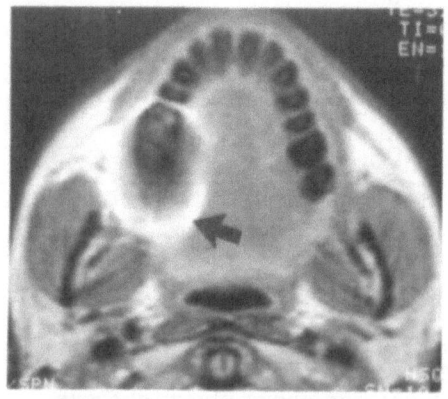

FIGURE 10
Artefact on MRI image due to dental filling.

REFERENCES

1 Fletcher RH, Fletcher SW, Wagner EH (1982) Clinical Epidemiology-the essentials. Williams & Wilkins, Baltimore.

2 Gademann G, Haels J, König R, Mende U, Lennarz Th, Kober B, Kaick G van (1986) Kernspintomographisches staging von Tumoren der Mundhöhle, des Oro- und Hypopharynx sowie des Larynx. Röfo 145: 503-509.

3 Gatenby RA, Mulhern CB Jr, Strawitz J, Moldofsky PJ (1985) Comparison of clinical and computed tomographic staging of head and neck tumors. AJNR 6: 399-401.

4 Hasso AN (1984) CT of tumours and tumour-like conditions of the paranasal sinuses. RadiologicClinics of North America, vol. 22, 1: 119-130.

5 Kondo M, Horiuchi M, Shiga H, Inuyama Y, Dokiya T, Takata Y, Yamashita S, Ido K, Ando Y, Iwata Y, Hashimoto S (1982) CT of malignant tumours of the nasal cavity and paranasal sinuses.Cancer 50: 226-231.

6 Lehman EL (1975) Nonparametrics: Statistical Methods Based on Ranks. Holden-Day Inc., San Fransisco.

7 Lund VJ, Howard DJ, Loyd GAS (1983) Evaluation of paranasal sinus tumours for cranio-facial resection. British Journal of Radiology 56: 439-446.

8 Maatman G (1986) High Resolution Computed Tomography of the paranasal sinuses, pharynx and related regions. Martinus Nijhoff Publishers Dordrecht.

9 Mancuso AA, Hanafee WN (1985) Malignant Sinus, Benign Sinus: chapter 1 and 2 from CT and MRI of the head and neck. Second edition, Williams & Wilkins, Baltimore.

10 Mees K, Vögl Th, Seiderer H (1984) Kernspintomographie in der Hals-Nasen-Ohrenheilkunde. Laryng. Rhinol. Otol. 63: 485-487.

11 Mödder U, Steinbrich W, Heindel W, Lindemann J, Brusis T (1985) Indikationen zur Kernspintomographie bei Tumoren des Gesichtsschädels und Halsbereiches. Digit. Bilddiag. 5: 55-60.

12 Sisson GA, Johnson NE, Amiri CS (1963) Cancer of the maxillary sinus: clinical classification and management. Ann. Otol. 72: 1050-1059.

13 Som PM, Biller HF, Lawson W, Sacher M, Lanzieri CF (1984) Parapharyngeal Space Masses: An Updated Protocol Based Upon 104 Cases. Radiology 153: 149-156.

14 Uhlenbrock D, Radtke J, Beijer HK, Machtens E, Pastoors H (1986) Ergebnisse der Kernspintomographie bei Tumoren des Gesichtsschädels.

   Röfo 144:322–327.

15 Ziedses des Plantes BG, Slegte RGM de, Gerritsen GJ, Sperber M, Valk J,
   Kaiser MC, Crezée FC, Snow GB (1987) Magnetic Resonance Imaging in
   malignant lesions of the paranasal sinuses. In print.

Acknowledgements
We want to thank Ms. Grace Roquas and Letty Bergfeld for their help in
preparing the manuscript.

CLINICAL   RELEVANCE   OF MRI   IN   THE   DIAGNOSIS   OF
DISEASES OF THE BRAIN.

O.J.S. Buruma

All scientific thinking is in terms of probability (Aldous
Huxley). This particularly pertains to the diagnosis of diseases.
Diagnosis is not an end in itself, but the starting point for thera-
peutic and prognostic considerations.
The question to adress here is what the relevance is of NMR for
improving the diagnosis of diseases of the brain in terms of probability.
In making a diagnosis in Neurology at least four levels of agre-
gation can be distinguished. These levels are
              - the functional diagnosis
              - the anatomical diagnosis
              - the histological diagnosis
              - the etiological diagnosis
The   functional   diagnosis   usually   is   the   outcome   of   careful
history taking and neurological examination, but it is no more
then a description of what is wrong in functional terms. Although
this first stage may be looked upon as being a mere transcription
(and usually translation into Latin or Greek) of the complaints
and visible restraints of the patient it has to be correct and
complete for the clinician to make the next diagnostic step.
This next step is the step towards the anatomical diagnosis.
A   thorough   examination   of   the   "neurological   patient"   usually
results in a package of abnormalities. These abnormalities have
to be arranged in such a way as to lead to a probable anatomical
diagnosis. Here again at least five possibilities exist. All
abnormalities can be explained by
              - one focal abnormality
              - one abnormal system (e.g. a cerebellar atrophy)
              - two or more abnormal systems (e.g. amyotrophic lateral
                sclerosis, subacute combined degeneration of the spinal
                cord).
              - diffuse abnormalities (e.g. metabolic encephalopathy)
              - multiple abnormalities (e.g. multiple sclerosis, multiple
                metastases)

The most intelligent thirteenth century monk Occam of Oxford has
already pointed out that it is much more attractive to explain
numerous observations by one cause than to postulate many causes
for one or few facts.
Be that as it may the classical brain imaging techniques nowadays
are there to help the clinician with his anatomical diagnosis.
These imaging techniques up till now have not been able to con-

tribute to a diagnosis at the level of histology with sufficient confidence to build on for further clinical decision making.
What about MRI and histology of diseases of the brain?
Soms authors feel inclined to state that MRI does contribute to the
histological diagnosis of diseases of the brain in a probabi-
listic manner. Such a statement, however, is much to inaccurate
to be of any use. If such statement is to mean anything at all it
has to be pinpointed to the type of lesion involved. Such statement for instance might well be true for a focal space occupying
lesion showing flow phenomena (aneurysm) but absolutely wrong for
any postulate about the histology of e.g. white matter disease.
In short if we are to discuss the diagnostic accuracy of MRJ in
terms of sensitivity and specificity for the histology of
diseases of the brain we have to define the type of disease at
stake.
To the best of my knowledge no studies prevail as yet presenting
such precise data on MRI and histology of diseases of the brain.
One should bear in mind that predictions about histology may have
far reaching consequences and in such cases should have a very
high probability to permit to abstain from further histological
or cytological verification.
Back therefore to the anatomical diagnosis in Neurology. Thinking
about MRI in terms of its contribution to Neurology one automatically
comes down to a comparison between MRI and CT-scan since CT-scan is
now widely available and centers with MRI but without CT will be few
if they exist at all.
I will confine myself here to the standard MRI imaging and leave
the most promising research on MRI spectroscopy with e.g. ^{31}P,
^{23}Na, ^{13}C aside. By standard MRI imaging I mean spin-echo and
inversion-recovery techniques without the use of paramagnetic
agents such as gadolinium or any other promising chemicals.
In general the resolution in MRI brain imaging is about the same as
that of X-ray CT but the soft tissue contrast of MRI is superior. One
of the most remarkable features of MRI imaging by spin echo techniques, however, is the unparalleled differentiation between grey and
white matter within the brain. Although modern CT-scan models do present us with some differentiation between grey and white matter, the
differences in attenuation are small. This gives NMR by far the lead
in detecting white matter disorders such as demyelinating diseases and
numerous infectious, postinfectious, metabolic, toxic, traumatic,
vascular and nutritional conditions in which either demyelination or
otherwise increased water content of the white matter is a prominent
feature. The effective differentiation of white and grey matter
further allows the neurologist to define relative degrees of white and
grey matter involvement in the disease process of the so-called degenerative diseases.This group encompasses the "selective cell death"
(or abiotrophic) syndromes, the mitochondrial encephalopathies and the
abnormal (lysosomal) storage syndromes. MRI is that sensitive in the
detection of white matter lesions that such lesions can be observed in
20 to 30 % of clinincally healthy elderly subjects. These lesions
usually appear to be of vascular origin.
This brings us to the most frequent group of neurological affections,
summarized under the heading stroke. The group of supratentorial
heamorrhagic strokes i.e. intracerebral, subarachnoid and
(spontaneous) subdural haemorrhage in general at present can better be

detected by CT than by MRI, but there is one study presenting two iso-
dense subdural haematoma's demonstrated by MRI but not visualized by
CT. This implies that the confirmation of the presence or absence of
intracranial haemorrhage, with the possible exception of supratentorial subdural haemorrhage, is not facilitated by MRI imaging. The
same applies to the detection of blood in haemorrhagic infarction.
With respect to supratentorial ischaemic stroke MRI appears to be able
to show infarction of the brain within less than 24 hours while CT is
still negative. For early ischaemic lesion detection MRI therefore is
clearly superior to CT. It is still too early to comment on the degree
of reversibility of these early abnormalities. For later stage
ischaemic lesions in general MRI probably is at least as sensitive as
and in many cases more sensitive than CT but exact figures of sensitivity and specificity are lacking. Ischaemic lesions in the region
of the sylvian fissure, of interest with respect to neurobehaviour can
much better be visualized by MRI because of the easy way of getting
coronal cuts and the absence of partial volume effects. The often
multiple small deep infarcts known as lacunar infarcts are better
visualized by MRI than by CT. This can be deducted from the fact that
in case of multiple lacunes MRI tends to demonstrate more lesions than
CT. With respect to arteriovenous malformations MRI is superior to CT
without the use of contrast because it is able to show the presence of
a fast flow of blood which emits almost no signal. If however such
malformation is suspected CT with contrast enhancement is probably
still best for confirmation of the lesion. If the use of contrast
medium is contra-indicated MRI however may be the alternative.
In supra tentorial tumors MRI in general is probably somewhat superior
to CT with contrast enhancement in detecting the lesion. This is especially true for primary neopolasms except some meningiomas. Metastases
and choleosteatomas are usually better visualized with CT.
With respect to the prediction of the histologic type of the lesion CT
and NMR probably yield comparable inaccurate information. The use of
intravenous gadolinium-DTPA probably results in enhancement in
cerebral metastases equal to, or even better than CT with contrast.
This allows for a good distinction between tumor and peritumoral
oedema, which may be difficult in MRI without the use of gadolinium.
Up till here I have confined myself to supratentorial brain pathology.
What has been said for the contents of the skull above the tentorium
of course also pertains to the posterior fossa. In the posterio fossa
however a strong supplementary advantage of MRI over CT is due to the
absence of beam hardening artefacts in MRI. With respect to the
brainstem another important additional advantage of MRI is the perfect
imaging of the sagittal and parasagittal planes. This makes MRI for
mass lesions in the cerebellopontine angle-petromastoid region and for
pathology of the brainstem and other structural lesions in the
posterior fossa undoubtedly the method of choice. The big advantage of
MRI over CT in not having any bone artefacts, on the other hand, forms
one of its disadvantages. MRI is inferior in showing pathology of the
skull itself and the demonstration of intracranial calcifications is
poor compared to CT. Bone changes involving the marrow containing
diploic space of the calvarial vault are usually more clearly
visualized.
In acute traumatology, where one is looking for signs of cerebral con-
tusion (besides oedema this means in essence blood) as well as skull
lesions there is at present no reason at all to switch from CT to

MRI.
MRI may show abnormalities in patients with partial seizures based on non-tumerous structural lesions localized by PET hypometabolism. It appears to be more sensitive than CT in this respect. MRI is superior to CT in detecting quitte a number of other more or less rare neurological abnormalities e.q. tuberous sclerosis, and many extrapyramidal disorders. In Parkinson's disease MRI may become a useful diagnostic tool by measuring the breadth of the pars compacta. The relevance of MRI for such disorders of course should not be measured by its impact on the world's health but by its relevance for the individual patient affected.
In summary MRI in general appears to be a bit more sensitive than CT in detecting supratentorial diseases of the brain, especially white matter disorders. MRI shows its virtues even more explicitly in the infratentorial region. This way MRI does add considerably to the diagnostic acumen of the neurologist at the level of the anatomical diagnosis. With respect to the histological diagnosis there still is no substitute for histology itself.

MRI OF THE SPINE: DEGENERATIVE DISC DISEASE AND INFECTION

A. DE ROOS, P.H.L. KESSING

INTRODUCTION
   Magnetic Resonance Imaging (MRI) is a sensitive modality to detect and
characterize abnormalities of the spine. MRI can detect abnormalities of
the disk and adjacent bone marrow in patients with degenerative disk disease (1). In a recent study the frequency and appearance of bone marrow
changes along the end-plates in degenerative lumbar disc disease were assessed (1).
   Normal vertebral bone marrow consists of hemopoietic marrow which demonstrates an intermediate signal intensity on MR images with both short
and long TR/TE pulse sequences (2). The normal lumbar vertebral body shows
an intermediate signal intensity on both short and long TR/TE pulse sequences due to the fatty component of the hemopoietic marrow. The normal
intervertebral disc demonstrates a relatively homogeneous low-signal intensity on short TR/TE pulse sequences, and the normal nucleus pulposus
shows an increased signal intensity with a central cleft on long TR/TE
pulse sequences. Disc degeneration results in decreased signal intensity
of the disc; in these cases the nucleus pulposus and annulus fibrosus can
become indistinguishable.
   Bone marrow changes adjacent to the vertebral end-plates can occur in a
variety of pathological conditions. On spinal MR imaging, we have observed
focal alterations in bone marrow signal intensity adjacent to the
end-plates in patients with degenerated discs.
   Increased signal intensity on the intervertebral disk can be helpful in
diagnosing disk-space infection on MR scans. Modic et al. (2) concluded
that MRI was more sensitive in detecting disk-space infection than either
conventional radiography or CT. It was as sensitive as radionuclide studies and more specific. Aguila et al. (3) showed that, in the absence of a
normal intranuclear cleft, an increased signal intensity of the disk is
suggestive of disk-space infection.
   One of the advantages of MRI is that it displays the infected nucleus
and the paravertebral extension in a single image. Furthermore, MRI does
not involve the use of ionizing radiation, making it well suited for repeated follow-up studies.

Degenerative Disc Disease
   Magnetic resonance studies of the lumbar spine in 41 patients were ana-
lyzed at 203 disc levels to assess the appearance and frequency of bone
marrow changes adjacent to normal and degenerated discs. At 58 out of 203
disc levels degenerative changes were found and in 29/58 (50%) of these
levels an abnormal bone marrow signal pattern was identified. On short
TR/TE pulse sequences, 24/58 degenerated discs showed an increased signal
intensity adjacent to the disc. In 17/24 changes were band-like on both
sides of the disc (Fig. 1);

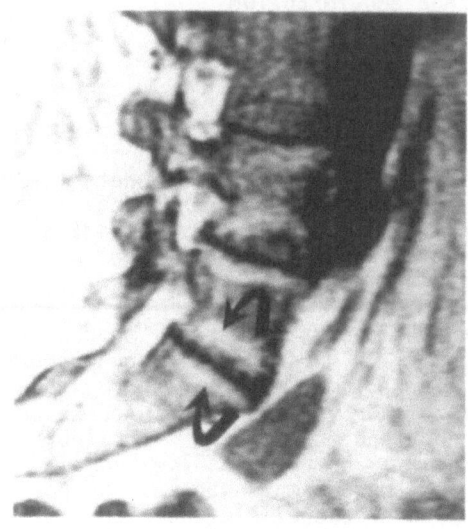

FIGURE 1.   Sagittal MR image (600/25)
              demonstrates band-like increased bone marrow signal on both
              sides of disc levels L4-L5 and L5-S1 (arrows).

in 4/24 a focal increase in signal on one side of the disc was found; the
remaining demonstrated a band-like and focal increase in signal on either
side of the disc. The relatively high signal intensity on short and long
TR/TE pulse sequences suggests fatty marrow conversion.

   At one degenerated disc, a band-like low signal intensity was observed
on both short and long TR/TE pulse sequences, which appeared to be related
to bony sclerosis. Four other degenerated discs demonstrated decreased
signal intensity on short TR/TE pulse sequences and high signal intensity
on long TR/TE pulse sequences. Conceivably these latter changes are due to
a local ischemic process with some inflammatory response. Recognition of
these marrow changes in degenerative disease is important in differentiating them from neoplastic or infectious disease involving disc-space and
adjacent end-plates. Furthermore, these focal marrow alterations may be
related to the pathogenesis of degenerative disc disease.

   Besides visualizing disc-space disease, MRI has also great potential in
diagnosing disc herniation (Fig. 2).

Spondylodiscitis

Infection is initiated in most cases by hematogenous spread of organisms, located first in the anterior aspect of the vertebral body near an intervertebral disk. The developing inflammatory process may erode the cortical bone, destroy the intervertebral disk, and involve the adjacent vertebral body. Subligamentous spread and paraspinal extension of tuberculosis is a frequent finding. Abscess formation is commonly bilateral, and small calcifications are characteristic of tuberculosis. Healing in tuberculous spondylitis can lead to partial or complete fusion of vertebral bodies. The lower thoracic and upper lumbar spine are predilection sites for tuberculosis.

The typical plain radiographic appearance of tuberculous spondylitis is

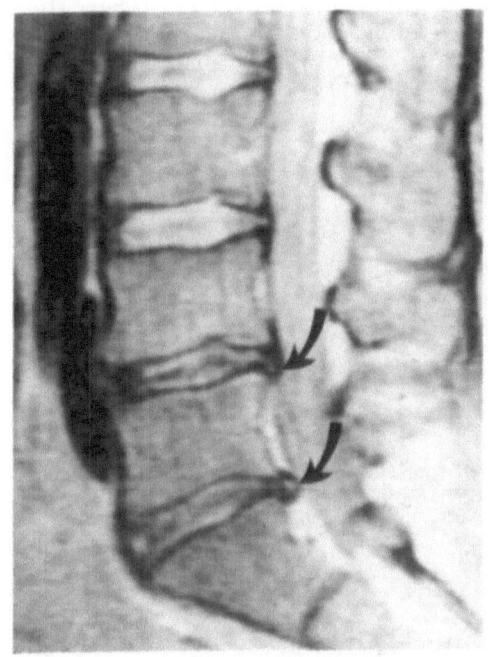

FIGURE 2.   Sagittal T2-weighted MR image
shows decreased signal intensity of degenerated disc levels
L4-5 and L5-S1.
Note small disc herniations at these levels (arrows).

irregularity of the vertebral end-plates, decreased height of the intervertebral disk, sclerosis of the surrounding bone, and in a later phase a
a tendency to anterior wedging of fusion.

Soft tissue extension and involvement of the spinal canal are well demonstrated by CT. Furthermore, CT is well suited to show abscess formation
as a mass with a low-density center and a definable wall, which becomes
clearer in enhanced CT scans.

Four patients with paravertebral extension of advanced tuberculous intervertebral disk-space infection were studied by CT and MRI (4). In one
patient gadolinium-DTPA (GD-DTPA) was administered intravenously as a paramagnetic contrast agent. MRI showed the disk-space abnormalities and
extension of the inflammatory process to best advantage in the coronal
plane. This plane demonstrated in one image the spinal localization and
the paravertebral extension of the inflammation. Gd-DTPA assisted in delineating the communication of the vertebral and paravertebral components
of inflammation (Fig. 3).

This phenomenon introduces an additional diagnostic element into the
evaluation of spondylitis. Although the features of advanced tuberculous
spondylitis are conspicuously well shown with MRI, further experience is
needed to evaluate the potential of MRI in detecting early tuberculous
spondylitis in relation to nontuberculous spondylitis.

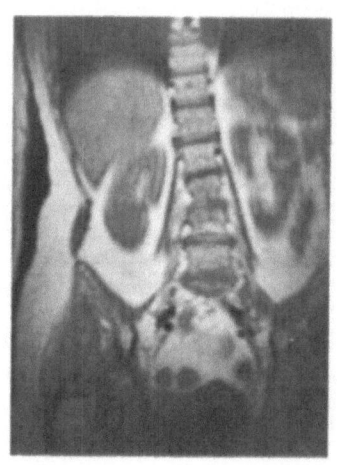 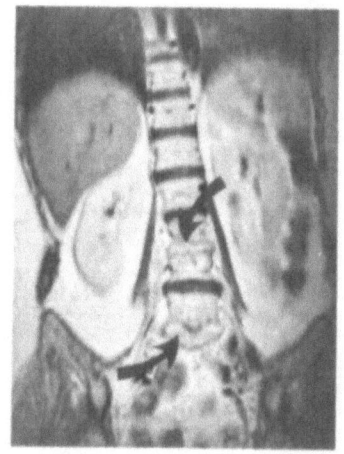

FIGURE 3.   Patient with spondylodiscitis at the lumbar level L3-4 and
              L5-S1.
          a) Coronal view of lumbar spine. Decreased height of disc level
             L3-4 is demonstrated.

          b) Coronal view of lumbar spine after intravenous injection of
             Gadolinium-DTPA (same imaging technique as in Fig. a).
             Note contrast enhancement at disc levels L3-4 and L5-S1 (ar-
             rows). Infected nucleus is now well demonstrated. In addi-
             tion, paravertebral abces information in the right psoas
             muscle is demonstrated to better advantage.

REFERENCES

1. De Roos A, Kressel H, Spritzer C. Dalinka M. Magnetic Resonance Imaging of End-Plate Marrow Changes in Degenerative Lumbar Disc Disease. AJR (in press).

2. Modic TM, Pavlicek W, Weinstein MA, et al. magnetic resonance imaging of intervertebral disk disease: clinical and pulse sequence considerations. Radiology 152: 103-111; 1984.

3. Aguila LA, Piraino DW, Modic TM, Dudley AW, Duchesneau PM, Weinstein MA. The intranuclear cleft of the intervertebral disk: magnetic resonance imaging. Radiology 155: 155-158; 1985.

4. De Roos A, Van Persijn van Meerten EL, Bloem JL, Bluemm RG. MRI of Tuberculous Spondylitis. AJR 146: 79-82; 1986.

MRI OF THE SPINAL CORD

G.M. Bydder

INTRODUCTION

The application of MRI to the spinal cord followed soon after its use in the brain. Indeed early papers often referred to MRI of the brain and cervical cord as a single entity. The initial studies with MRI recognised both advantages and disadvantages (1,2). In these studies gross lesions, Arnold Chiari malformations and most cases of syringomyelia were recognised, but the resolution of MRI images was limited and the future for MRI in the spinal cord appeared less than that in the brain. All this was changed by the use of surface coils.

By using simple saddle or planar coils closely applied in turn to the cervical, thoracic and lumbar spine, image quality was radically improved. Now there appears to be little doubt that MRI is the technique of first choice for disease of the spinal cord. It has the advantage that the use of an intrathecal contrast agent is not required. In addition, detail of the spinal cord is revealed directly rather than indirectly as a filling defect on myelography.

The scope of MRI has been further extended by the use of the intravenous contrast agent Gadolinium-DTPA (Gd-DTPA) (3) and the application of new pulse sequences to the detection of CSF flow.

In practical, clinical terms MRI of the lumbar spine is one of the commonest MRI examinations now performed and an excellent book describing the technique and the principles of image interpretation in this region has recently appeared (4).

TECHNIQUE

A surface coil adapted to the particular area of the spine is essential and a variety of possible designs have been described (5). It is usual to divide the spinal column into three segments and examine these separately.

This corresponds in general clinical terms to the types of clinical problems referred but not infrequently it is necessary to include two or more 'segments' of the spinal cord leading to long examination times.

While artefacts are not usually a problem, they may arise from respiratory movements in the neck, thorax and abdomen as well as CSF flow. The use of surface coils tends to minimise the effect of respiratory movements and various forms of bipolar or more complex gradient pulses such as MAST (Motion Artefact Suppression Technique) can be used to reduce the effect of CSF movement (6).

In general the sagittal plane is usually chosen as the orientation of choice with transverse images used especially for disc disease. The coronal plane is sometimes of value and oblique slices are especially useful for demonstrating the intervertebral foramena.

The choice of pulse sequence depends on machine capability but in general a T_1 dependent spin echo has been used to display the margins of the cord. This sequence is also useful for syrinx and cystic lesions. In order to demonstrate lesions within the cord T_2 weighted spin echo sequences have been used. At higher fields these sequences provide a higher signal intensity for CSF than for brain producing a myelographic effect. This is useful in the diagnosis of extramedullary disease.

The inversion recovery sequence displays high T_1 dependent contrast. The spinal cord normally appears narrower with this sequence than with SE sequences. More recently the partial saturation (PS) sequence has been used with a reduced flip angle in order to increase the speed of the examination.

IMAGE INTERPRETATION

T_1 dependent sagittal images provide an excellent basis for assessing cord size. It is also the technique of choice for assessing anatomical detail at the craniovertebral junction. In general this sequence is valuable for displaying fluid cavities, but if these contain protein or breakdown products from hemorrhage, the contrast difference may be low.

Abnormal regions are usually highlighted on T_2 dependent spin echo sequences, but care is necessary in diagnosing lesions when the CSF signal is greater than that of the normal cord because lesions may be simulated by partial volume effects.

The PS sequence is more prone to movement and metallic artefacts and displays chemical shift effects in the vertebral bodies. The PS sequence is generally more sensitive to the paramagnetic breakdown products of hemaglobin than corresponding spin echo sequences with the same values of TR (repetition time) and TE (echo time).

SYRINGOMYELIA

What previously seemed a relatively unusual condition is now seen very frequently with MRI. The 'classical' syrinx is a straightforward diagnosis (Fig. 1) although thin slices are to be preferred in making the diagnosis and it is always possible that a syrinx may be collapsed at the time of examination. Transverse scans may be more helpful here. Complex syrinxes with mixed solid and cystic components and an irregular appearance can present a more difficult problem in diagnosis. The lesion may be a syrinx alone or it may be a syrinx associated with a tumor. Alternatively the diagnosis may be a tumor with a cystic component. Gliosis alone may increase T_2 so the presence of a high signal intensity area at the margin of a syrinx does not necessarily help in diagnosis.

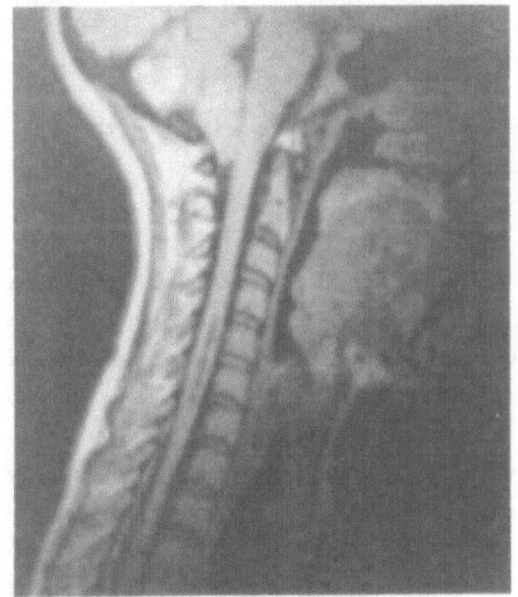

FIGURE 1. Syringomyelia: SE544/44 scan. The syrinx has a low signal intensity.

In this situation enhancement with Gd-DTPA (intravenous) may be used to indicate likely tumor involvement although absence of enhancement does not exclude tumor (Fig. 2).

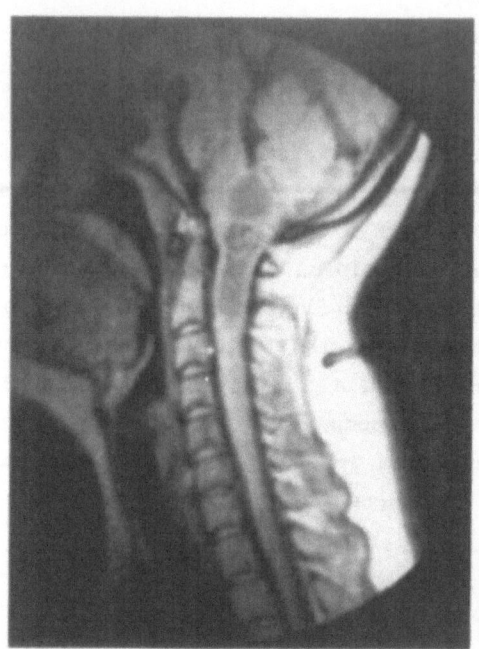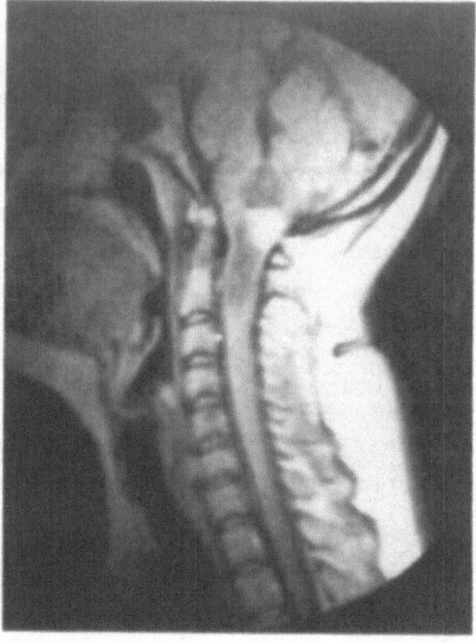

FIGURE 2.   Hemangioblastoma: SE544/44 scans a) before and b) after I.V. Gd-DTPA.   The small region of tumor enhances.

TUMORS (8)

Expansion of the cord is the sine qua non for diagnosis of an intrinsic tumor although other lesions may expand the cord.   Generally there is an increase in T_1 and T_2. The association with cyst is common, and separation between tumor and edema may be difficult although this is sometimes dramatically improved with Gd-DTPA. The usual 'myelographic' rules apply to the diagnosis of extramedullary tumors. The fact that they frequently show strong contrast enhancement is also of value (Fig. 3).

DISC DISEASE (4,9,10)

This is common and can usually be recognised with MRI. The principles of interpretation are similar to those with CT, and the book by Steinmetz (4) mentioned previously provides a systematic guide to interpretation.

The significance of degenerative changes may be difficult to assess. The working rule is that non-degenerative discs do not herniate though there may be exceptions to this in the acute situation and in young patients.

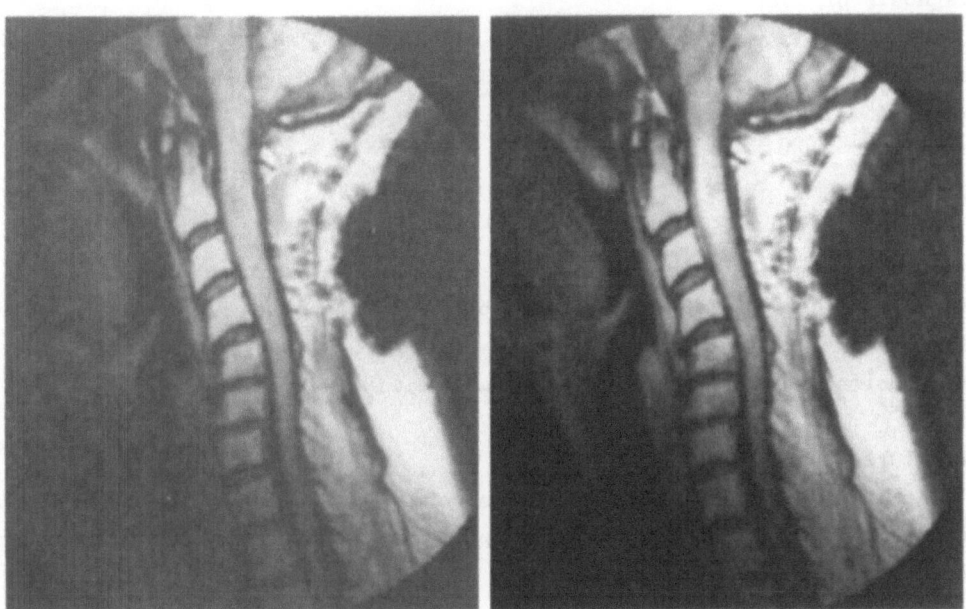

FIGURE 3. Metastatic tumor from the nasopharynx: SE544/44 scans a) before and b) after I.V. Gd-DTPA. The area of tumor enhances within the expanded cord.

TRAUMA

Encroachment in the spinal canal by bone is reasonably well displayed with MRI. Fractures can be seen, as can hemorrhage, within and around the cord. Late sequelaes such as atrophy, cyst formation or syringomyelia are well shown although myelomalacia can present difficulties.

CONGENITAL LESIONS (11)

Craniovertebral anomalies are well displayed. In pediatric practice lipomas, tethered cord and varying degrees of myelomeningocele have been demonstrated. The Arnold Chiari syndromes were described early on in the development of MRI and remain a common reason for referral.

DEMYELINATING DISEASE, TRANSVERSE MYELITIS

Silent MS plaques are not so common in the spinal cord as they are in the brain and often the clinical imperative is to examine the brain in a patient with a spinal cord lesion in order to establish or refute the diagnosis of MS.

Transverse myelitis of multiple etiology is well shown. It may be associated with some expansion of the cord, raising the possibility of tumor. A follow up examination may be indicated here.

INFECTION

Overt bacterial or viral infection in the cord, subarachnoid, subdural or adjacent spaces has been described and visualised with MRI. The fluid collection has a long T_1 T_2 in cases of abscess. Diagnosis may be difficult in cases of focal myelitis where it is possible to demonstrate the abnormal region but not provide a specific diagnosis.

ARTERIOVENOUS MALFORMATIONS (8)

Dephasing with the spin echo sequence can be used to demonstrate vascular patterns and the PS sequence can be used to demonstrate any associated hemorrhage.

CONCLUSION

The progress of MRI in both the brain and spinal cord has been remarkable. MRI emphasizes the unity of the CNS by not requiring any great change of technique between the brain and spinal cord.

The ability to replace myelography with MRI is a major advantage. It obviates the need for hospitalisation and a lumbar puncture as well as the possibility of an early or late reaction to the contrast agent.

Much work is now being performed on CSF studies although the clinical impact has been limited to date. Other developments which include the use of fast scanning techniques (PS, etc) are progressing, but already MRI offers a great deal in this region of the body.

REFERENCES

1. Modic MT, Weinstein MA, Pavlicek W, et al: Magnetic resonance imaging of the cervical spine: Technical and clinical observations. AJR 141: 1129-1136, 1983

2. Norman D, Mills CM, Brant-Zawadski M, et al: Magnetic resonance imaging of the spinal cord and canal: Potential and limitations. AJR 141: 1147-1152, 1983

3. Bydder GM, Brown J, Niendorf HP, Young IR: Enhancement of cervical intraspinal tumors with intravenous gadolinium-DTPA. J Comput Assist Tomogr 9(5): 847-851, 1985

4. Steinmetz ND: MRI of the Lumbar Spine: A Practical Approach to Image Interpretation. Slack, New Jersey, 1987

5. Bydder GM, Butson PR, Harman RR, Gilderdale DJ, Young IR: Use of spherical receiver coils in magnetic resonance imaging of the brain. J Comput Assist Tomogr 9(2): 413-414, 1985

6. Pittany F: Motion artefact suppression technique. J Comput Assist Tomogr (in press)

7. Di Chiro G, Doppman JL, Dwyer AJ: Tumors and arteriovenous malformations of the spinal cord: assessment using MR. Radiology 156: 689-697, 1985

8. Gibson M, Buckley J, Mawhinney R, et al: Magnetic resonance imaging and discography in the diagnosis of disc degeneration. Nottingham, England: Journal of Bone and Joint Surgery 68-B:3 369-373

9. Modic MT, Masaryk T, et al: Lumbar herniated disk disease and canal stenosis: Prospective evaluation by surface coil MR, CT and myelography. AJNR 7: 70901-717, 1986

10. Barnes PD, Lester PD, et al: Magnetic resonance in infants and children with spinal dysraphism. AJNR 7: 465-472, 1985

MRI in occult spinal dysraphism.

G.J.Vielvoye(1),R.A.C.Roos(2) and P.H.L.Kessing(1).

Department of Diagnostic Radiology,subdivision of
Neuroradiology(1) and the department of
Neurology,subdivision of Child Neurology (2),
University Hospital Leiden,
Leiden,The Netherlands.

The term spinal dysraphism is first used by Lichtenstein(1)
to describe disorders in all tissue layers of the back.Both
the overt and the occult spina bifida are included.The overt
variant,including the meningocele and the meningomyelocele
are easily recognized immediately after delivery.
The occult form,including
diastematomyelia,diplomyelia,dermoid cyst and sinus,lipoma
and lipomeningomyelocele are much more difficult to
diagnose.
The age of manifestation varies between birth and 15
years,but an onset in adults has also been described (2).In
our series the latest onset of symptoms was seen in a 63
years old patient.
The clinical syndrome is often summarized as the tethered
cord syndrome,independant of the causing factor (3).The
syndrome comprises slowly progressive
neurological,orthopaedic and urological symptoms often in a
combination.Insidious changes in gait,muscle weakness of the
legs,irradiating pain,differences in leg lenght,bladder
disturbances and primary or secundary incontinence may be
the first symptoms (4).
The occult spinal dysraphism is often combined with a big
variety of clinacal signs as hypertrichosis,naevus,dermal
sinus or scarring.Often their are combinations with
abnormalities at the level of the cranio-cervical
junction.The Arnold-Chiari malformation is the most common
one.
In the past the diagnosis tethered cord was confirmed with
myelography.Computerized tomography added important
information.Especcially the relation of fatty tissue,in case
of a lipoma,to the dural sac can be determined with CT
(5-7).
Since MRI came available in our department,we prefer this
diagnostic tool in case of tethered cord syndrome.Without
agressive techniques information is obtained about the
length and shape of the spinal cord,the localization of
fatty tissue in case of a lipoma and the shape of the
vertebral column and spinal canal.A risky lumbar puncture in
an anatomical abnormal area can be avoided with MRI.
A 0.5 tesla Gyroscan is used in combination with a surface

coil,applicated in the lumbar or cervical region.A set of
T1,proton density and strongly T2 weighted sagital sections
is obtained with the spin-echo technique.The T1 images give
information about the spinal cord,the proton density
pictures and strongly T2 weighted images learn us about the
CSF and the soft tissue wich surround the spinal cord.

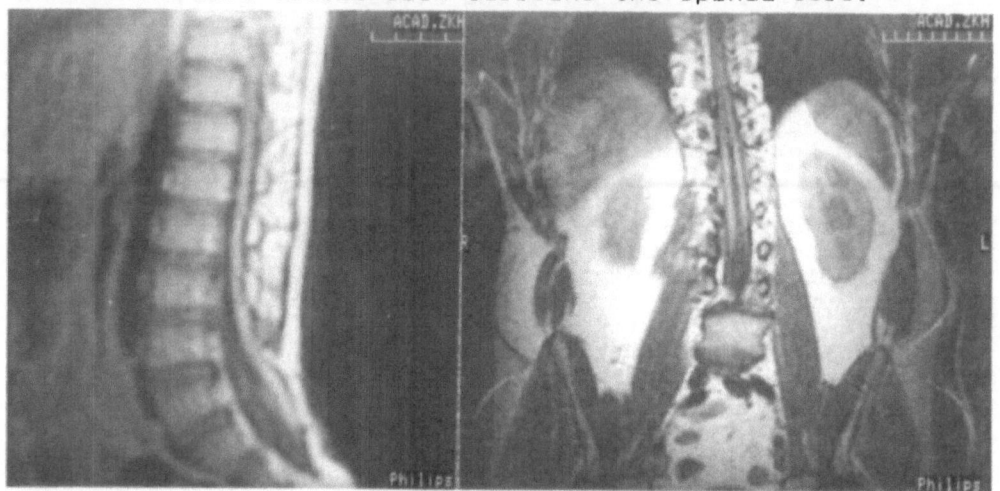

The T1 weighted sagittal section demonstrates a malascensus
of the spinal cord and arc defects in the sacral region.The
coronal scan shows a diplomyelia.

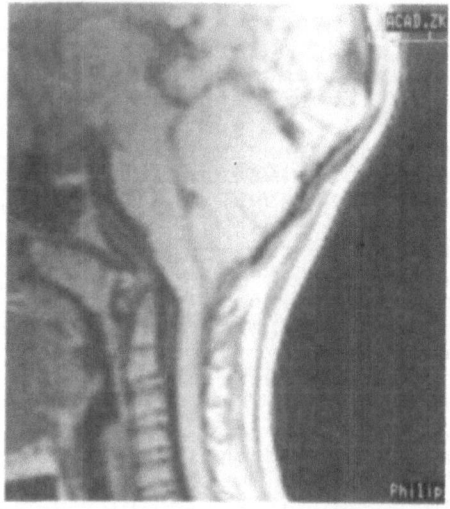

At the level of the cranio-cervical junction an Arnold
Chiari malformation can be observed.The cerebellar tonsils
are below the level of the foramen magnum.

References:
1:Lichtenstein,B.W.1940,Spinal dysraphism.Arch Neurol

Psychiat 44:792
2:Pang,D.,Wilberger Jr,E,1982,Thethered cord syndromes in
the adults.J Neurosurg 57:32.
3:Till,K.1968,Spinal dysraphism:a study of congenital
deformations of the back.Dev Med Child Neurol 10:470
4: Bakker-Niezen,S.H,De gekluisterde conus of tethered
spinal cord,thesis Nijmegen,1986.
5:Gryspeerdt,G.L.1963,Myelographic assesment of occult forms
of spinal dysraphism.Acta Radiol Diagn 1:702
6:Fritz,C.R,Harwood-Nash,D.C,1975,The tethered conus.Am J
Roentgenol Radium Ther Nucl Med 125:515.
7:James,HE,Oliff,M,1977,Computer tomography in spinal
dysraphism.J Comp Assist Tomogr 1:391.

CLINICAL RELEVANCE OF MRI
IN DISEASES OF THE SPINE AND CORD

J.H.C. VOORMOLEN

1. HISTORY

Magnetic Resonance Imaging (MR) offers the neurosurgeon an extra dimension in diagnostic imaging. In the beginning there was the X-ray of the vertebral column and the bony structures were detected. In combination with intrathecally located contrast medium a nice view in the sagittal plane of the contours of the spinal cord (myelography) and the cauda (caudography or saccography) were obtained and enormously appreciated. After some years more details of the anatomic and pathologic spine and spinal cord were made visible by means of the CT, but the value was limited by the transverse plane. Than came the MR and a new world was opened. In the sagittal plane the "whole" spinal cord was imaged. Moreover, the cord itself and the pathologic process in the cord were visible! Without the harm of irradiation! Besides these "open doors", what is the clinical relevance of MR?

2. RELEVANCE
2.1. Which diagnosis? Without being exhaustive you can see the neurological diagnoses that can potentially benefit from MR in Table 1. Nearly all diagnoses can be made with MR. In this table, the diagnoses that are now preferably imaged with the MR are underlined. But few MR apparatus are available and investigations are time consuming, so the question is for which diagnosis offers MR better information than other neuroradiological imaging techniques.

2.2. Better information is information that leads to a more detailed diagnosis, or a more accurate localisation of the pathological process, but, as well, information that can be obtained with much lesser burden for the patient. The clinical relevance of MR in diseases of the spine and spinal cord is only significant if MR provides better information in this sense. I should like to introduce to you three patients.

2.3. Patients
2.3.1. The first patient, a female born in 1976, presented in april 1985 with a clinical history of pain in the neck and right arm since january 1985. There were three periods of progression of tetraparesis during fever. Neurologically, the lesion should be located over a long section of the cervical spinal cord because of the flaccid paresis without tendon reflexes in both arms. Severe pain in neck and arms suggested

TABLE 1

ETIOLOGY DYSFUNCTION OF THE SPINAL CORD

1 extradural	2 extramedullary	3 intramedullary
1.1 tumor	**2.1** tumor	**3.1** tumor
vertebral metastasis chordoma vertebral hemangioma aneurysm. bonecyst primary bone tumor plasmacytoma lipoma eosinof. granuloma giant cell tumor	meningioma schwannoma neurofibroma epidermoid lipoma neurenteric cyst	astrocytoma ependymoma hemangioblastoma teratoma epidermoid lipoma metastasis mixed tumor
1.2 vascular	**2.2** vascular	**3.2** vascular
epidural hematoma	subdural hematoma AVM	AVM infarct
1.3 degenerative	**2.3** degenerative	**3.3** degenerative
spondylosis herniated disc * rheumatoid arthritis (C1-C2 slip)		syringomyelia hydromyelia atrophy of cord
1.4 infectious	**2.4** infectious	**3.4** infectious
spondylitis discitis epidural empyema	meningitis subdural empyema	myelitis schistosomiasis abscess
1.5 trauma	**2.5** trauma	**3.5** trauma
vertebral luxation vertebral fracture	root avulsion	root avulsion
1.6 congenital	**2.6** congenital	**3.6** congenital
narrow canal bony spurs diastematomyelia	tethered cord meningocele	tethered cord Chiari malf, myelomeningocele

* cervical herniated disc with cord compression.

MR preference underlined.

involvement of the roots. The fever pointed to an infection. The MRI made a tumor more likely. The MR showed that the lesion extended over a long section but a tumor was not clearly depicted. Some kind of misunderstanding between the neuroradiologist and the neurosurgeons concerning the interpretation of

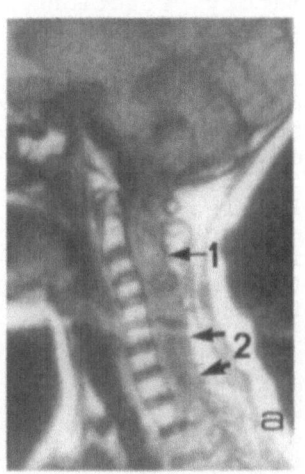 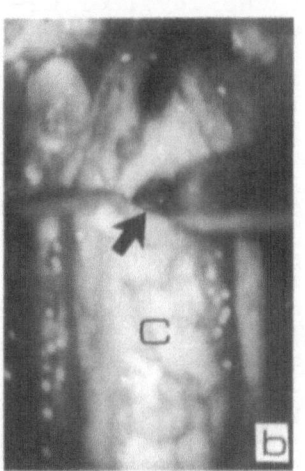

FIGURE 1. a) Patient 1, preoperative MRI (0.5 T, TR 250 ms, TE 30 ms) arrow 1: first operation (white spot), arrow 2: second operation (area of low signal intensity). b) Patient 1, intraoperative view of the abnormal tissue on the place of the biopsy (arrow) at C2-C3 at the first operation, C: spinal cord.

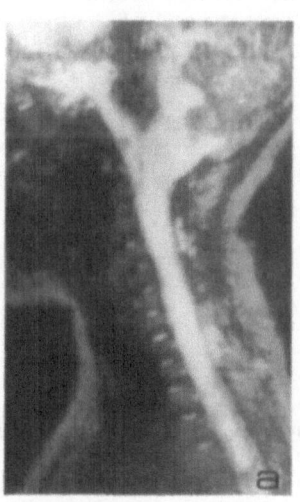 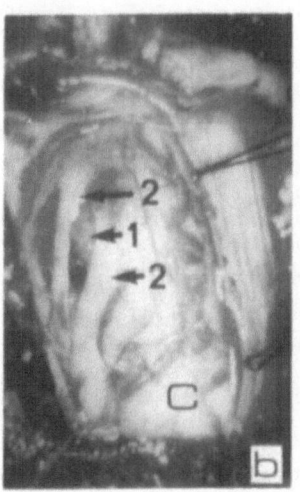

FIGURE 2. a) Patient 1, preoperative MRI (0.5 T, TR 1000 ms, TE 50 ms) extension tumor from medulla oblongata to D 5. b) Patient 1, second operation at C7-D1, intraoperative view, arrow 1: tumor, arrow 2: roots, C: spinal cord.

the MR led to the first operation that turned out to have been
unnecessary. The operation was directed to the white spot on
the MRI (Fig. 1a). The surgeon thought that bleeding occurs in
the tumor, but the pathological anatomy showed that they can
also occur in a necrotic area. In the biopsy (April 29, 1985)
taken at the level of C2-C3 an inflammatory reaction without
tumor cells was seen. At operation, it was obvious that the
cord was swollen and rotated (Fig 1b).
The combination of inflammation and possible lymphoma cells in
the CSF led to a period of intensive investigation for systemic
tumors, lymphomas and infections. In the meantime, the neurological status of the patient deteriorated. The second operation
(May 14, 1985) did show the tumor (Fig. 2b). Now the operation
was directed to the area of low signal emission in the lower
cervical cord that could be seen on the first preoperative MRI
(Fig. 1a). The extend of the tumor is depicted on the MRI,
nicely (Fig. 2a). This knowledge (extension from medulla
oblongata to D5) changed the policy of surgical decompression
followed by radiotherapy to radiotherapy alone. This policy
proved to be successful.
We did learn from this case that solid tumors in the cord are
not always so nicely depicted as tumors with cysts. Treatment
policies should be tuned to the individual patient. MRI helps
to provide a base for decisions. Especially the border of the
tumor in the lower brain stem will be difficult to establish
with the conventional imaging techniques.
Interpretation of MRI may be very difficult. One should take
into account the scanning parameters. This process of learning
to know what you see is only possible if the neurosurgeon takes
the time to listen to the neuroradiologist. But the neuroradiologist should teach the neurosurgeon and others how the
different parameters influence the depiction of the tissue.
Only clinicians who have learnt this can be partners in the
discussion with (neuro)radiologists.

2.3.2. The second patient, a boy was born in 1969 with a flaw
on the back. He started to walk later as his sister and became
completely continent at the age of 12 years. When he was 14
years old he became secondary incontinent followed one year
later by a slight paresis of his right leg. MRI showed
tethering of the spinal cord. The cord terminates in a lipoma.
There is no cauda (Fig. 3a).
In that time we performed a myelogram (Fig. 3b) in combination
with CT to make the diagnosis. To introduce the contrast agent
a lumbar puncture has to be performed with the risk of
puncturing the spinal cord that lies very dorsally in this kind
of patients. MR is much less hazardous for the patient and can
be performed being an outpatient. The CT with intrathecally
located contrast shows the CSF, the cord and the lipoma (Fig.
4a). Once you have got the pictures the diagnosis is not
difficult but the risks to get the pictures are much higher
than with MRI. We gained 1,5 cm for the untethering of the cord
(Fig. 4b).

2.3.3. The third patient, a female born in 1938, has
rheumatoid arthritis and suffered pain in the neck for one

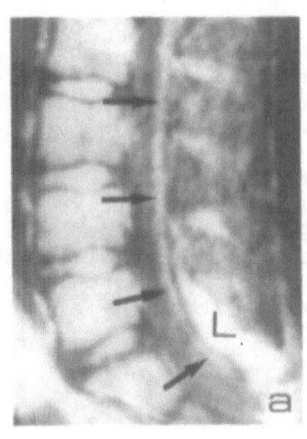
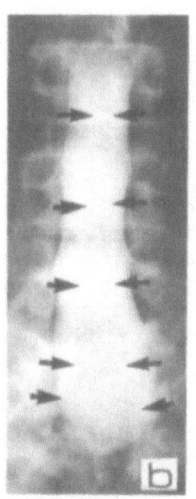

FIGURE 3. a) Patient 2, preoperative MRI (0.5 T, TR 1000 ms, TE 150 ms) arrows: dorsally located spinal cord terminates at vertebra S2. L: lipoma. b) myelogram with metrizamide, arrows: lipoma with spinal cord.

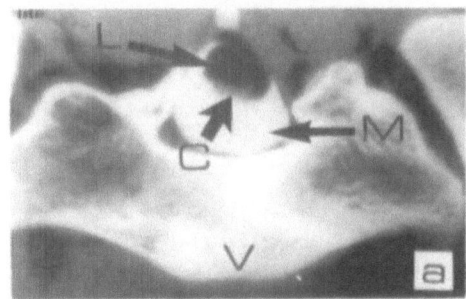
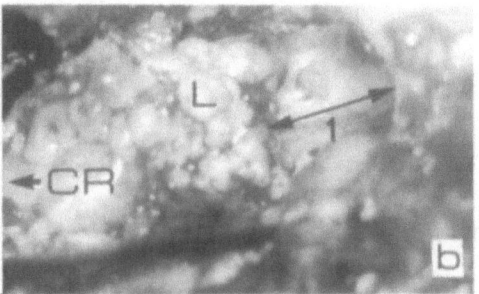

FIGURE 4. a) Patient 2, preoperative CT with metrizamide. V: ventral, M: metrizamide in CSF, C: spinal cord, L: lipoma. b) Patient 2, intraoperative view. CR: cranial, L: lipoma, l: distance of untethering (1.5 cm).

year. The neck became gradually more stiff and more flexed. At last neurological symptoms appeared. In rheumatoid arthritis often an erosion of the odontoid process of axis occurs by the inflammatory process. Sometimes this leads to instability in the cranio-cervical junction. The fact that the X-ray showed a deformity did not surprise (Fig. 5a). When you want to do something for the patient then you need to know exactly where the compression is and how many segments are involved.

I agree that a planigram can give you more information. But never the information that the MRI gives you (Fig. 5b). The combination of depicting the nervous tissue and the bone in one picture is unique for the MRI. Taking into account the difficulty in performing a cervical myelogram in this painful group of patients mostly because of the inability to extend the neck properly makes the MRI an enormous step forwards for these patients. In this patient there was a compression of the lower brain stem and of the spinal cord (Fig. 6a and 6b). This situation gives considerable problems in deciding how to decompress the nervous tissue and restore stability. We judged this kind of "data acquisition" so important that we removed a skull traction unit made of iron and replaced it after the MRI. These small operative procedures are a lesser burden for this kind of patients than a combination of myelography and CT.

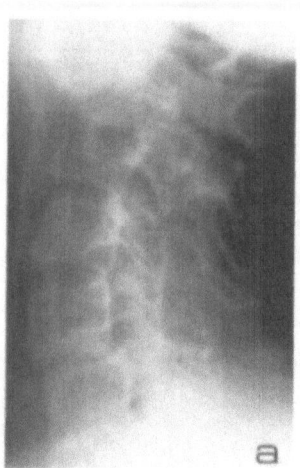 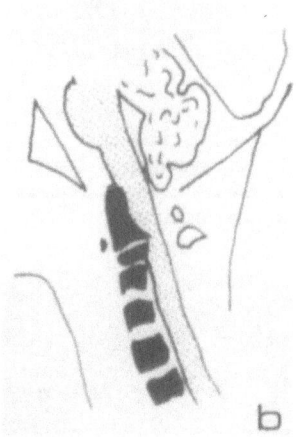

FIGURE 5. a) Patient 3, preoperative X-Cervical spine. b) Patient 3, drawing of the information from MRI.

2.4. Comments

2.4.1. Tumor. It is obvious that most progress has been achieved in the diagnosis of the intramedullary tumors. In this area all other imaging techniques failed. An important fact is that in the glioma group the tumor extends often over significant more segments than the surgeon thought using the information of a myelogram only. In some cases failure to benefit from the operative procedure could be ascribed to incomplete removal or incomplete decompression of the spinal cord due to tumor in the not-operated segments. Cysts in the cord are more frequently diagnosed with MR. Sometimes it appeared difficult to differentiate between tumor cysts and syringes. Nowadays, with more experience, few misinterpretations occurred.

2.4.2. Vascular lesions. In these rare disorders I would like to draw your attention to the infarcts. In the first stages when the diagnosis is not yet made and the symptoms are alarming the MR can show you edema of the cord. Anyway, the absence of a tumor or compression can make the diagnosis more likely.

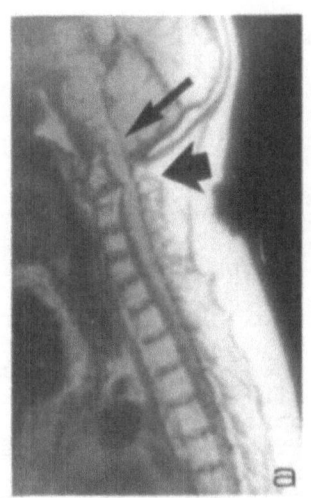 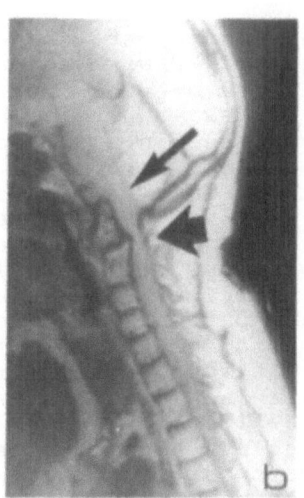

FIGURE 6.   a) Patient 3, preoperative MRI (0.5 T, TR 550 ms, TE 30 ms), arrows: site of compression of the brain stem and spinal cord. b) Patient 3, preoperative MRI (0.5 T, TR 2000 ms, TE 50 ms), arrows: site of compression of the dura covering the brain stem and spinal cord.

2.4.3. Degenerative lesions. It is beyond doubt that more cases of syringomyelia will be diagnosed in the near future. I mean this in the neuroradiological fashion. I expect a lot of cavities filled with various amounts of fluids will be seen on MR scans. To correlate these cavities with a clinical syndrome may be difficult. Probably a large heterogeneity exists in this group of syndromes and research will have to select clinical entities that might be eligible for surgical treatment. For the diagnosis of spinal cord compression in the cervical region MR is excellent. It is possible to differentiate between compression of the dura and compression of the cord itself. Moreover, information about the degree of degeneration of the intervertebral disc is obtained from the same scan. In this way the information is collected that could have been provided only by a combination of myelography and discography in a former era. The lesser burden and pain for the patient is clear.

2.4.4. Congenital lesions. This group of patients benefits in two ways from the MR. The sagittal plane offers the opportunity to follow the pathological process from cervical to sacral. It is easy to determine a malascensus of the cord, and to name the corresponding vertebra. The risk of introduction of contrast through or into the cord is avoided, using the MR technique. To complete this, the information provided to the surgeon is much more detailed and accurate. Cavities are well delineated. The filum terminale is often visible. Fat tissue or epidermoid tumors can be anticipated.

3. FUTURE

The near past showed us how many improvements in the technique of MR were accomplished in a couple of years. Recent improvements are the application of surface coils and the pulse gated images to avoid loss of signal due to CSF pulsations. Both resulted in a substantial improvement of the details in the images of the cord.

With this fact in mind it is hard to believe that one of my wishes will not be realized in the near future. The vertebral column has several curvatures. Most MR scans that are now available use straight slices. This means that only in per-fectly straight columns a full sagittal picture can be obtai-ned. Many patients do have some degree of scoliosis. Currently, it is possible to use a reformation of the data to compute an image that follows the curvatures of the vertebral column. This results in an image that shows the whole cord in one picture in one plane (e.g. through the central canal in a frontal plane). The trouble is that it costs a lot of time. A better solution might be to collect the data in a plane, that should be defined beforehand on the guidance of anatomical landmarks, indicated by the radiologist in one segment, and than computed by the apparatus in an analogous way for the other segments.

4. CONCLUSION

To conclude my assay of the clinical relevance I must confess that MRI is a real improvement in diagnosing disorders of the spinal cord and the spine. The neurosurgeon gets a more accurate localisation of the lesion, that may lead to a better diagnosis. It is beyond any doubt that the burden for the patient is significantly reduced.

Let there be more MR-apparatus!

Acknowledgment.
The technical assistance with the illustrations was provided by Mr. G.J. van de Giessen.

SECTION III CARDIOVASCULAR IMAGING

IDENTIFICATION OF SEGMENTAL CARDIAC ANATOMY USING MR IMAGING

GERARD L. GUIT, JOHN ROHMER

INTRODUCTION

Reports have shown that the use of electrocardiographic gated magnetic resonance (MR) imaging may provide high-quality images in patients with congenital heart disease (1, 2).

To establish the potential of MR imaging with regard to the demonstration of segmental cardiac anatomy, we obtained MR images from 20 patients with levotransposition of the aorta.

This abnormal relation of the great arterial vessels is present in different congential heart diseases, such as congenitally corrected transposition, complete transposition, univentricular hearts and double-outlet ventricles.

Though the relation of the great arterial vessels in these cardiac malformations may be the same, the atrioventricular and ventriculoarterial connections are different. In this chapter, we discuss the results obtained when the segmental approach is applied to MR imaging in this patient group. We will briefly consider the potential role of MR imaging in the clinical evaluation of other congenital cardiac diseases.

MATERIAL AND METHODS

We obtained MR images from 20 patients, two females and 18 males, who ranged in age from 9 to 50 years (Table 1).

Case No.	age (yr)/ Sex		Situs	Main Diagnosis
1	11	/ M	solitus	Corrected Transposition
2	12	/ M	solitus	Corrected Transposition
3	14	/ M	solitus	Corrected Transposition
4	17	/ F	solitus	Corrected Transposition
5	17	/ F	inversus	Corrected Transposition
6	22	/ M	solitus	Corrected Transposition
7	27	/ M	solitus	Corrected Transposition
8	29	/ M	inversus	Corrected Transposition
9	50	/ M	solitus	Corrected Transposition
10	16	/ M	solitus	Tricuspid Atresia
11	17	/ M	solitus	Double inlet left ventr.
12	19	/ M	solitus	Double inlet left ventr.
13	23	/ M	solitus	Double inlet left ventr.
14	23	/ M	solitus	Double inlet left ventr.
15	26	/ M	solitus	Double inlet left ventr.
16	29	/ M	solitus	Double inlet left ventr.
17	33	/ M	inversus	Double inlet left ventr.
18	42	/ F	solitus	Double inlet left ventr.
19	9	/ F	solitus	Complete Transposition
20	11	/ M	solitus	Double outlet R. ventr.

TABLE I. SUMMARY OF DATA ON PATIENTS WITH LEVOTRANSPOSITION OF THE AORTA

Identification of Segmental Cardiac Anatomy by Magnetic Resonance Imaging. A study in patients with Levo-Transposition of the aorta.

In all patients, levotransposition of the aorta and associated defects were demonstrated by angiocardiography. Thus we were aware of the anatomic diagnosis before the MR studies were performed. The Gyroscan system (Philips, the Netherlands) at our institution operates at 0.5 Tesla. A multiplanar approach (transverse, coronal, sagittal) was applied to imaging, and images were obtained using the two-dimensial Fourier transformation. During this study the matrix size was 128 x 128. Spatial resolution was 2.5-3.5 mm. The spin-echo pulse sequence was used with an echo time of 30 msec. Multisection packages contained five to eight adjacent sections that were 5-10 mm thick. In each series, four signal averages were obtained. Total examination time in each case varied form 40 to 70 minutes. In each case, the MR images were evaluated with respect to the visceroatrial situs, the ventricular morphology, the great arteries and their interrelationship, the atrioventricular connection, the ventriculoarterial connection and associated cardiac anomalies.

RESULTS
Examinations performed in 19 patients showed clear delineation of the internal cardiac structure, which permitted a detailed segmental analysis and evaluation of associated anomalies. In the remaining patient (case 14), poor image quality was obtained as a result of the patients irregular heart rhythm. This case was excluded from further study. The segmental analysis is demonstrated in cases involving congenitally corrected transposition (Figure I) and double inlet left ventricle (Figure II).

Identification of visceroatrial situs
The location of the morphologic right atrium (MRA) and the morphologic left atrium (MLA), atrial situs, was deduced from visceral situs in all patients. Coronal images depicted all the important anatomic features with respect to the diagnosis of situs, such as central bronchial anatomy and the positions of the inferior vena cava, the abdominal aorta, the liver, the spleen and stomach. Central bronchial anatomy could not be demonstrated on sagittal and transverse images.

Localization of the ventricles
Eleven patients had two normally developed ventricles(excluding those patients with a univentricular heart). In nine of the eleven cases, the level of attachment of the septal leaflets was identified; in ten of the eleven cases, the septomarginal trabecula was identified; in eight of the eleven cases, the trabecular pattern was identified; and in ten of the eleven cases the infundibulum was identified. Identification of these features allowed localization of the ventricles in all eleven cases. Compared with images obtained in the transverse plane, those obtained in the sagittal and coronal planes provided less information with respect to the identification of the ventricular morphology.

Localization of the great arteries
The aorta was identified in all patients by demonstrating its continuity with the aortic arch and brachiocephalic vessels. The pulmonary trunk was identified in all cases by demonstrating its continuity with the pulmonary arteries. The aorta originated left and anterior to the pulmonary trunk in situs solitus and right and anterior to the pulmonary trunk in situs inversus.

Atrioventricular connection
We directly identified the type of atrioventricular connection that was present in all cases by linking the atrial and ventricular segments together. The AV connection was concordant in one case, discordant in eleven cases, and a univentricular atrioventricular connection was present in eight cases (double inlet; 7; absence of the right AV connection; 1).
The univentricular connection was established by demonstrating that both atria were aligned with one ventricular chamber. In all cases, the main ventricular compartment communicates with a small ventricular chamber through a large ventricular septal defect. All of these small chambers were anterosuperior in location and were connected with the ascending aorta. The main ventricular chambers displayed a smooth wall that was compatible with a left ventricular pattern. These findings were consistent with a diagnosis of double-inlet left ventricle.

Ventriculoarterial connection
We directly assessed the type of ventriculoarterial connection that was present in each case by linking the ventricular segment and the great arteries together. This connection was discordant in 18 cases. In case 20 a double outlet connection was present.

Additional anomalies
We were able to identify the presence of additional cardiac abnormalities, such as ventricular septal defects (nine), infundibular pulmonary stenosis (two), as well as confirming various surgical results.
In two cases a persistent left superior vena cava was noted; this had not been identified prior to the performance of the MR studies.

DISCUSSION
The current study was designed to establish the potential role of MR imaging in depicting segmental cardiac anatomy among patients with recognized complex atrioventricular and ventriculararterial connections.
The morphology of the main bronchi and the location and relation of the inferior vena cava and the abdominal aorta are valuable indicators of atrial situs (3, 4, 5). These structures were readily identified on coronal images obtained through the thoracic and upper abdominal cavity. In this respect, MR imaging appears to possess relative advantages over echocardiography. When the latter imaging modality is used, the morphologic right and left atria are identified by their connections to the systemic and pulmonary veins; these criteria permit a determination of situs in the majority of cases (6). In patients with abnormal situs and anomalous venous connections, however, these criteria are not appropriate, and various complementary imaging modalities have been applied to establish atrial situs accurately. Conventional tomography is used to demonstrate bronchial anatomy (4), whereas colloid scintigraphy (7) and computed tomography (5) have been valuable in demonstrating abdominal anatomy. In our opinion, cardiac MR imaging is the first method that demonstrates all relevant anatomic structures; thus situs and the status of the spleen can be assessed without performing additional diagnostic procedures.
Transverse images are the most helpful in differentiating ventricular morphology, as they show the attachment of the septal leaflets to the septum, the septomarginal trabecula, the infundibulum, and the pattern of trabeculation. In univentricular hearts, the anterosuperior position of the rudimentary chamber and the smooth-walled appearance of the main

chamber convinced us that this ventricle was the morphologically left ventricle. Identification of the great arteries was achieved in all three planes.

Our results indicate that MR imaging depicts segmental cardiac anatomy in detail. Thus, MR imaging may be a valuable, noninvasive tool that can be used to analyze complex congential cardiac diseases, especially in those patients in whom the results of ultrasound examinations are not conclusive. Images can be obtained in every desired plane, while image acquisition is not restricted by the configuration of the thoratic cage or interposition of lung as in ultrasound studies. Immobilization of infants during image acquisition still is a problem in MRI.

In our experience MR imaging also has proved to be a valuable method in the evaluation of pulmonary atresia with ventricular septal defect, re-coarctation of the aorta, situs abnormalities, cardiac malpositions, and evaluation of the left ventricular outflow tract in atrioventricular sep-tal defects.

Acknowledgment: the authors wish to thank G. Kracht for photographical work and Fokje Noorderijk for manuscript preparation.

REFERENCES
1. Didier D., Higgins C.B., Fisher M.R., Osaki L., Silverman N.M., Cheitlin M.D. Congenital heart disease: gated MR imaging in 72 patients. Radiology 1986; 158: 227-235.
2. Higgins C.B., Byrd B.F., Farmer D.W., Osaki L., Silverman N.H., Cheit-lin M.D. Magnetic resonance imaging in patients with congenital heart disease. Circulation 1984; 70: 851-860.
3. Van Praagh R. The importance of segmental situs in the diagnosis of congenital heart disease. Seminars Roentgenol. 1985; 20: 254-271.
4. Partridge J.B., Scott O., Deverall P.B., Macartney F.J. Visualization and measurement of the main bronchi by tomography as an objective indica-tor of thoratic situs in congenital heart disease. Circulation 1975; 51: 188-196.
5. Tonkin I.L., Tonkin A.K. Visceroatrial situs abnormalities: sonographic and computed tomographic appearance. AJR1982; 138: 509-515.
6. Gussenhoven E.J., Becker A.E. Congenital heart disease: morphologic echocardiographic correlation. Edinburgh: Churchill Livingstone, 1983.
7. Fitzer P.M. An approach to cardiac malposition and the heterotaxy syndrome using Tc sulfur colloid imaging. AJR 1976; 127:1021-1025.

Figure I. MR images used in the segmental analysis of congenitally
corrected transposition involving situs solitus.
(a-d). Contiguous transaxial images.
(a). The septomarginal trabecula crosses from the septum to the
anterior wall of the posterior left-sided ventricle.
(b). The septal leaflet of the left AV valve attaches more
anteriorly to the septum than the septal leaflet of the right AV
valve, indicating that the left-sided is the tricuspid valve.
(c). The outflow tract of the posterior left-sided ventricle has
a completely musculur infundibulum.

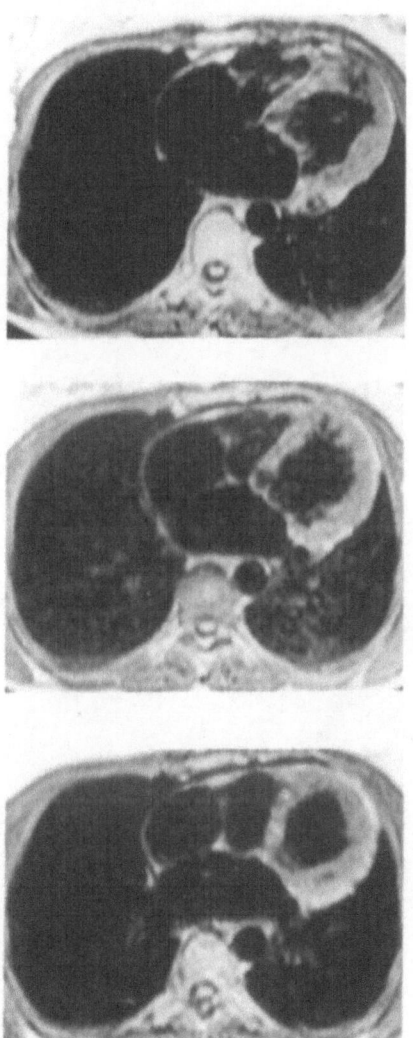

(d). Coronal image. The left ascending aorta originates from the left-sided ventricle.
(e). Sagittal image. The pulmonary trunk arises posterior to the aorta from the right-sided ventricle. Note anterior recess in front of the outflow tract to the pulmonary trunk.
(f). Oblique sagittal image. Supraventricular crest between the aortic and left-sided AV valve.

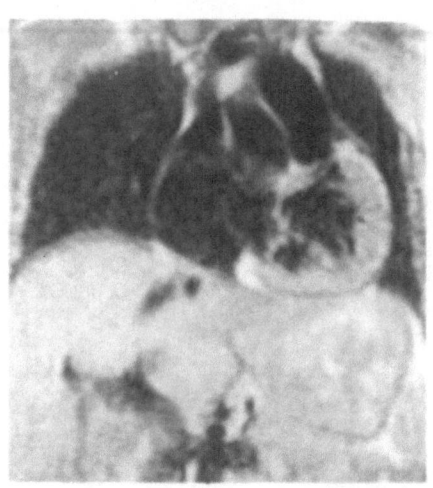

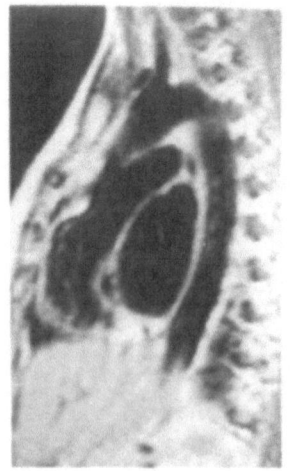 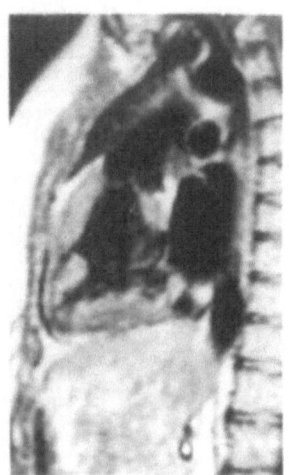

Figure II. MR images used in the segmental analysis of double inlet left ventricle involving situs solitus.
(a-c). Contiguous coronal images.
(a). The ventricular segment is divided by the septum into a main and a small compartment.
(b). The right atrium communicates with the main compartment. A small antero-superior located outlet chamber gives rise to the aorta. Both ventricular compartments communicate through a large septal defect.
(c). Left atrium also communicates with the smooth walled main ventricular chamber.

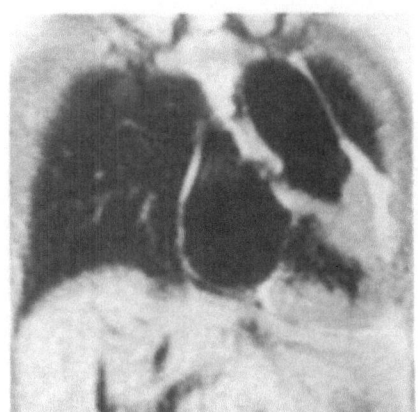
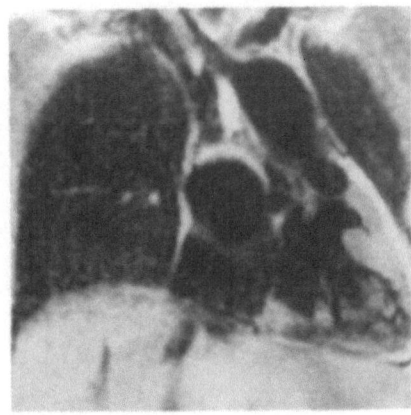

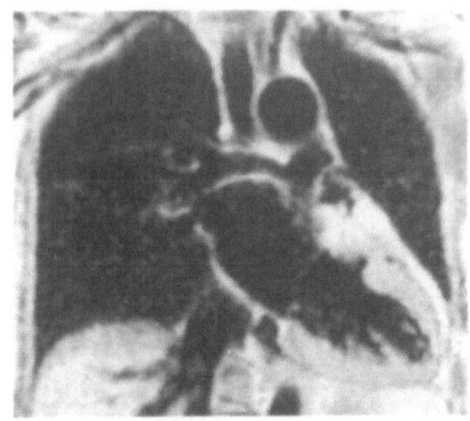

(d). Sagittal image demonstrates severe infundibular pulmonary stenosis.
(e). Transverse image. The large ostium of the aorta is left and anterior to ostium of the pulmonary trunk.

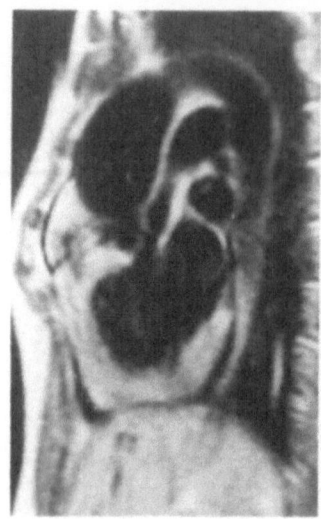

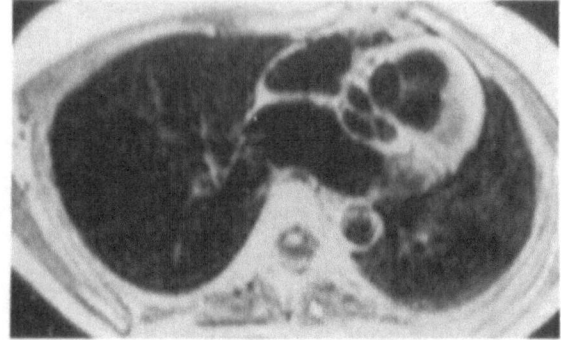

GATED MRI VERSUS ECHOCARDIOGRAPHY FOR EVALUATION OF CONGENITAL CARDIAC MALFORMATIONS.

MURRAY MAZER

INTRODUCTION

Gated magnetic resonance cardiac imaging can delineate congenital cardiovascular abnormalities in a noninvasive manner without requiring contrast medium or ionizing radiation (1-19). High-resolution two-dimensional echocardiography, however, has already established itself for such a purpose (20-27). Precatheterization echocardiography provides highly accurate evaluation of congenital cardiac malformations to better plan the subsequent cineangiographic projections, thus minimizing catheter manipulation, avoiding excess radiation and reducing contrast volume. In selected lesions, such as atrial septal defect, hypoplastic left heart syndrome and critical aortic stenosis in infancy, detailed echocardiography coupled with an understanding of the natural history and surgical alternatives can eliminate the need for preoperative catheterization. More detailed comparison of 2D-echocardiography and MRI of congenital cardiac malformations than previously has been reported is therefore necessary to better assess the relative advantages of each imaging discipline in the context of specific congenital cardiac lesions and management alternatives.

MRI Versus Echocardiography: General Comparisons

There are several general advantages of MRI over echocardiography. First there is a greater ability to transport a signal through air or bone than with echocardiography. There is therefore no limitation of view through the sternum and no hindrance to imaging in the presence of pneumomediastinum, pneumothorax, nor emphysema. Adult congenital heart disease in particular is not always easy to evaluate with echocardiography since the presence of an ossified sternum and a greater degree of substernal air produce limitations on traditional echocardiographic projections. Furthermore, without significant attenuation of signals by increasing distance from the energy source, resolution of remote structures deep within the body is unimpaired with MRI, unlike ultrasonography. An additional advantage of MRI over echocardiography is the wider field of view in the older child and teenager, with comparable spatial resolution. Thus, the right ventricle and pulmonary artery branches can be identified more completely, unlike the evaluation of older patients with echocardiography in whom these structures frequently cannot be evaluated as well due to "piecemeal" imaging. In addition, MRI provides improved great vessel and central pulmonary artery visualization as well as gross assessment of coronary arteries. Finally, visceroatrial situs, atrioventricular, and ventriculoarterial connections may be delineated in complex congenital heart disease in a more definitive manner with MRI in situations where echocardiographic analysis is inconclusive.

Conversely, there are several general disadvantages of MRI as compared to echocardiography. First the installation and maintenance costs are very expensive and contribute to the high patient cost. Second, imaging time to produce satisfactory signal-to-noise ratios is considerably longer for MRI. However, continuing improvement in early, prototype MRI equipment may ameliorate this temporary disadvantage as faster imaging techniques appear

to be emerging on the horizon. Certainly, there is a greater potential for
image degradation from body motion and rapid and deep respiration with MRI
than echocardiography. Therefore, more patient cooperation and possible
sedation may be necessary. Unlike echocardiography, true real-time imaging
is not possible at present with MRI, and evaluation of valvular function
is limited. However, more dynamic "fast-field echo" imaging using a combination of gradient reversal echoes and small flip angles is being
introduced that will allow some easier identification of regurgitant jets
and shunts (28).

Combined echocardiographic-Doppler studies provide an estimated pressure
gradient in valvular lesions whereas comparable information is not possible as yet with MRI (although there may be a potential for quantitation
of blood flow by MRI) (29-32). In the critically ill infant and child the
presence of support equipment such as monitoring devices, pacing apparatus, and oxygen supply all present a ferromagnetic interference that pro-
hibits the MRI study entirely. Improved shielding by manufacturers in the
future may negate this disadvantage. Portable studies at the bedside are
not possible with MRI. The presence of arrhythmias negates the advantages
of ECG-gating. Finally, there is a 2 to 5 percent incidence of claustrophobia encountered in the early clinical experience with MRI. Future MRI
improvements with better spatial resolution of a 512x512 matrix, faster
imaging and patient throughput, functional evaluation with dynamic MRI,
flow-study quantitative analysis and spectroscopic metabolic assessment
are all on the horizon. Some of these "breakthroughs" in technological
advancement will occur and some may not, similar to the evolution of TC
scanning over the last decade.

Nevertheless, the relative simplicity of echocardiographic equipment
compared to that for MRI and the numerous additional above-mentioned
echocardiography advantages make it the obvious noninvasive imaging procedure of choice for most congenital cardiac malformations.

It is therefore not as important to assess the accuracy rate for MRI of
lesions that echocardiography already images very well. To better assess
the role for MRI of congenital cardiac malformations it is more important
to assess what it images better than, rather than equal to, echocardiography. Therefore, a more detailed evaluation of the early cases in our
series with echocardiographic and MRI comparisons provided the following
analysis of the main potential for MRI in this field (33):

MRI versus Echocardiography: Specific Comparisons

1) Global assessment of the right ventricular outflow tract, right
ventricular wall thickness and especially pulmonary artery developments
were consistently better with MRI than echocardiography in patients with
right heart obstructive disease. After the initial echocardiographic
and/or angiographic diagnosis of Tetralogy of Fallot, pulmonary atresia,
or tricuspid atresia, follow-up MRI prior to definitive surgery may negate
the need in some patients for additional preoperative cardiac catheterizations.

2) Sinus venosus ASD that is frequently difficult to assess by echocardiography was only noted by MRI. The associated partial anomalous right
upper lobe pulmonary vein draining to the SVC can also be identified by
MRI better than echocardiography, when angled views are utilized.

3) Differentiation between a very large VSD, where a small septal rem-
nant may still provide the foundation for surgical repair, and a single
ventricle where a surgical attempt to separate it into the two ventricles
is less likely, was felt to be more definitive with MRI. Some muscular

VSD's in the lower ventricular septum were better appreciated noninvasively with MRI.

Evaluation of the bulboventricular foramen defect in complex congenital heart disease is frequently more definitive with gated MRI than echocardiography.

4) Aortic arch anomalies and adjacent great vessel takeoffs were consistently more clearly assessed with MRI in older children and adults where echocardiographic windows frequently are suboptimal. There is a real potential for MRI assessment of coarctatation (along with complimentary echocardiograhy of intracardiac anatomy) to negate the need for preoperative intravenous digital subtraction angiography or selective intraarterial angiography in this lesion entirely. The critical coarctation interrupted arch and truncus anomalies of infancy may, however, still require catheterization for definitive assessment, while maintaining critical monitoring and support devices during the imaging procedure.

5) A persistent left SVC draining to the coronary sinus was visualized only by MRI (although the dilated coronary sinus on echocardiography did indirectly point to its presence). While this lesion is potentially visualized with echocardiography, the important presurgical information of relative size of the right and left SVC and the presence or absence of an intercommunicating left innominate vein are more easily obtainable (short of catheterization) by MRI than echocardiography.

6) Blalock-Taussig and Waterston shunt evaluation was superior with MRI rather than echocardiography. Follow-up evaluation of shunt patency with MRI could obviate catheterization follow-up in some cases.

7) Patency of Rastelli and Fontan conduits after repair of severe right ventricular outflow tract narrowings and tricuspid atresia were better appreciated by MRI and could obviate some follow-up catheterizations.

Incorporation of a right ventricular conduit into the sternotomy defect was noted only by MRI, and could be a significant anatomical finding should reoperation be necessary.

8) Patency of repaired anamalous pulmonary venous return that has been reanastomosed into the left atrium and diversion of systemic and venous channels in Mustard and Senning correction of D-TGV's were better assessed by MRI and could obviate some follow-up catheterizations. In a prospective controlled evaluation of 15 such postoperative patients MRI was highly sensitive and exceedingly specific for detecting both superior and inferior limb narrowings following intra-arterial repair of transposition of the great arteries as compared to both contrast and pulsed Doppler echocardiography (34).

9) Finally, complex cases of visceroatrial situs abnormalities above and below the diaphragm were better assessed by MRI. In general, the more complex the congenital heart disease the more gated cardiac MRI has to offer.

On the other hand, pulmonary, aortic and subaortic valvar stenosis were generally not adequately identified by MRI as compared to echocardiography (with the exception of one adult pulmonary valvar stenosis). Distal hilar left pulmonary artery occlusive changes were also missed by MRI. This latter abnormality should be visualized with MRI and warrants further study with axial and/or obliquely angulated views since echocardiography is seldom helpful in this situation.

Conclusion

The role of MRI in the clinical evaluation of patients with congenital malformations is still undefined. Our study was limited to older patients and most of those examined by MRI had a known anatomic diagnosis established by angiocardiography and/or echocardiography. A prospective study with no knowledge of the diagnosis would better assess the true efficacy of MRI. On the other hand, it is quiet likely that most lesions to be examined by MRI will have prior echocardiography and, hence, an established clinical diagnosis.

Even though anatomical spatial resolution of congenital heart disease is frequently superior with gated MRI than with echocardiography, it is unlikely that MRI will replace echocardiography as the simplest and most definitive method of establishing a noninvasive diagnosis in patients with congenital cardiac malformations. MRI is more likely to become a complimentary additive noninvasive imaging procedure to answer some questions left in doubt by echocardiography (mainly extracardiac artery and vein assessments) and as a preferred follow-up following imaging method in certain clinical circumstances such as postoperative temporary shunt and permanent conduit evaluations.

Angiocardiography will remain necessary to provide vital physiological data, i.e., chamber-pressures, shunt volumes, oxygen saturations, and pulmonary vascular resistance. However, MRI can negate some follow-up catheterizations in appropiate clinical circumstances, and the tendency for congenital heart disease evaluation to become more and more noninvasive will continue. The potential for MRI evaluation of noninvasive blood flow measurements (29-32), tissue characterization (35-37), and even myocardial metabolism assessment (38-39) is intriguing and awaits further clinical evaluation.

REFERENCES
1. Herfken RJ, Higgins CB, Hricak H, et al. Nuclear magnetic resonance imaging of the cardiovascular system: normal and pathological findings. Radiology 1983; 147: 749-759.
2. Higgins CB, Stark D, Mc Namara M, et al. Multiplane magnetic resonance imaging of the heart and major vessels: studies in normal volunteers. AJR 1984; 142: 661-667.
3. Lieberman JM, Alfidi RJ, Nelson AD, et al. Gated magnetic resonance imaging of the normal and diseased heart. Radiology 1984; 152: 465-470.
4. Fletcher BD, Jacobstein MD, Nelson AD, et al. Gated magnetic resonance imaging of congenital cardiac malformations. Radiology 1984; 150: 137-140.
5. Jacobstein MD, Fletcher BD, Nelson AD, et al. ECG-gated nuclear magnetic resonance imaging: appearance of the congenitally malformed heart. Am Heart J 1984; 107: 1014-1020.
6. Higgins CB, Byrd BF III, Farmer DW, et al. Magnetic resonance imaging in patients with congenital heart disease. Circulation 1984; 70(5): 851-860.
7. Didier D, Higgins CB, Fisher MR, et al. Congenital heart disease: Gated MR imaging in 72 patients. Radiology 1986; 158: 227-235.
8. Dinsmore RE, Wismer GL, Guyer D, et al. Magnetic resonance imaging of the interatrial septum and atrial septal defect. AJR 1985; 145: 697-703.
9. Jacobstein MD, Fletcher BD, Goldstein S, et al. Evaluation of atrioventricular septal defect by magnetic resonance imaging. Am J Cardiol 1985; 55: 1158-1161.
10. Didier D, Higgins CB. Identification and localization of ventricular septal defects by gated MRI. Am J Cardiol 1986 (in press).
11. Jacobstein MD, Fletcher BD, Goldstein S, et al. Magnetic resonance imaging in patients with hypoplastic right heart syndrome. Am Heart J 1985; 110: 154-158.
12. Peshock RM, Parrish M, Fixler D, et al. MR imaging in the evaluation of the single ventricle. Radiology 1985; 157(P): 355.
13. Soulen RL, Donner RM. Advances in noninvasive evaluation of congenital anomalies of the thoracic aorta. Radiol Clin N Am 1985; 23: 727-736.
14. Glazer HS, Gutierrez FR, Levitt RG, et al. The thoracic aorta studied by MR imaging. Radiology 1985; 157: 149-155.
15. Von Schuulthess GK, Hiagashino SM, Higgins SS, et al. Coarctation of the aorta: MR imaging. Radiology 1986; 158: 469-474.
16. Fletcher BD, Jacobstein MD. MRI of congenital abnormalities of the great arteries. AJR 1986; 146: 941-948.
17. Fletcher BD, Dearborn DG, Laakman RW, Clampitt ME. MR imaging in infants with airway obstruction: Preliminary observations. Radiology 1986; 160: 245-249.
18. Jacobstein MD, Fletcher BD, Nelson AD, et al. Magnetic resonance imaging: evaluation of palliative systemic-pulmonary artery shunts. Circulation 1984; 70: 650-656.
19. Soulen RL, Donner RM. Magnetic resonance imaging of rerouted pulmonary blood flow. Radiol Clin N Am 1985; 23: 737-744.
20. Tajik AJ, Seward JB, Hagler DT, et al. Two dimensional realtime ultrasonic imaging of the heart and great vessels: technique, image orientation, structure identification and validation. Mayo Clin Proc 1978; 53: 271-303.
21. Henry WL, Maron BJ, Giffith JM. Cross-sectional echocardiography in

the diagnosis of congenital heart disease: identification of the relation of the ventricles and great arteries. Circulation 1977; 56:
267-273.

22. Allen HD, Goldberg SJ, Ovitt Tw, Goldberg BB. Suprasternal notch
echocardiography: assessment of the clinical utility in pediatric
cardiology. Circulation 1977; 55: 605-612.

23. Silverman NH, Snider AR. Two-dimensional echocardiography in congenital heart disease. Norwalk, CT: Appleton-Century-Crofts, 1982.

24. Goldberg SJ, Allen HD, Sahn DJ. Pediatric and adolescent echocardiography - a handbook. Year Book Medical Publishers, Inc., Second Edition, Chicago, 1980.

25. Weyman AE. Cross-sectional echocardiography. Philadelphia: Lea and
Febiger, 1982.

26. Bierman FZ. Two-dimensional echocardiography and its influence on
cardiac catheterization. Cardiovasc Intervent Radiol 1984; 7: 140-153.

27. Sahn DJ. Two-dimensional echocardiography as an aid to planning cardiac catheterization. Cardiovasc Intervent Radiol 1984; 7: 154-155.

28. Feiglin DHI. Gated cine MRI reveals congenital cardiac defects. Diagnostic Imaging, October 1986; 98-101.

29. Morse O, Singer JR. Blood velocity measurements in intact subjects.
Science 1970; 170: 440-442.

30. Kaufman L, Crooks LE, Sheldon P, Rowan W. Evaluation of NMR imaging
for detection and quantitation of obstructions in vessels. Invest Radiol 1982; 17: 554-560.

31. Crooks LE, Sheldon P, Kaufman L, Rowan W. Quantification of obstruction in vessels by nuclear magnetic resonance (NMR). IEEE Trans Nucl
Sci 1982; 29: 1181-1185.

32. Mills CM, Brant-Zawadzki M, Crooks LE, et al. Nuclear magnetic resonance: principles of blood flow imaging. AJR 1984; 142: 165-170.

33. Sandler MP, Graham TP, Mazer MJ, et al. Magnetic resonance imaging of
congenital cardiac abnormalities. Nuclear Medicine Annual 1986;
141-160.

34. Campbell RM, Moreau GA, Mazer MJ, et al. Detection of caval obstruction by MRI following intra-atrial repair of transposition of the
great arteries. Am J Cardiol (in press).

35. Higgins CB, Herfkens R, Lipton MJ, Sheldon P, Kaufman L, Crooks LE.
Nuclear magnetic resonance imaging of acute myocardial infarctions in
dogs: alterations in magnetic relaxation times. Am J Cardiol 1983; 52:
184-188.

36. Herfkens RJ, Sievers R, Kaufman L, et al. Nuclear magnetic resonance
imaging of the infarcted muscle: a rat model. Radiology 1983; 147:
761-764.

37. Wesbey G, Higgins CB, Lanzer P, Botvinick E, Lipton MJ. Imaging and
characterization of acute myocardial infarction in vivo using gated
nuclear magnetic resonance. Circulation 1984; 69: 125-130.

38. Jacobus WF, Taylor GI, Hollis DP, et al. Phosphorus NMR of perfused
working hearts. Nature 1977; 26: 756-760.

39. Nunally RL, Bottomley PA. 31P NMR studies of myocardial ischemia and
its response to drugs. J Comput Assist Tomogr 1981; 5: 296.

CLINICAL RELEVANCE OF MRI IN CONGENITAL ABNORMALITIES OF THE CARDIOVASCULAR SYSTEM

J. ROHMER

To evaluate the nature and the severity of congenital heart defects, the clinician can, next to the patient's history and findings on physical examination, use simple techniques like electrocardiography and routine X-ray examination of the chest. Although providing valuable information, seldom if ever do these investigations yield sufficient information to allow important decisions to be taken, like the decision whether or not to operate. Of the many additional methods available for further refinement of the cardiac diagnosis, the two most informative - cardiac catheterization/angiocardiography and echo/Doppler-cardiography - will be compared to each other and to MRI (1). On the basis of this comparison a tentative recommendation for the use of MRI in cardiovascular diagnosis of congenital heart disease will be given.

In many instances cardiac catheterization combined with selective angiocardiography remains the most accurate and complete diagnostic method for the evaluation of patients with congenital heart diease, providing the most complete image of the abnormal anatomy and its functional sequelae. It is, however, an invasive method using contrast medium and submitting both patient and investigator to X-ray radiation. It is time-consuming, lasting one to three hours. Young children have to be heavily sedated or anesthetized. The intervention can only be performed in a specialized X-ray laboratory with expensive equipment and personnel.

Echo/Doppler-cardiography is a non-invasive method that can be applied at the bedside or even when the patient is in an incubator. It does not use ionizing radiation and can be repeated as often as is necessary. A complete study usually does not last longer than one hour. However, sedation often cannot be avoided. The method supplies anatomic as well as functional information in such plentiful detail that one often can refrain from cardiac catheterization and angiocardiography. This is especially advantageous in severely ill neonates.

Both methods can be used when the patient is connected to monitoring equipment or to an artificial ventilator. They provide instantaneous beat-to-beat information. However, echo/Doppler-cardiography images show only relatively small parts of the heart in each section, while sections of the heart and directions of flow measurements often cannot be obtained in the plane that would show the anomaly to its best advantage. Structures close to the sternum and close to the vertebral column can often not be clearly visualized. Especially in postoperative patients there often is a poor "echo-window". Modern echo/Doppler-equipment is certainly expensive, but much less so than a sophisticated catheterization laboratory. It also requires less personnel.

MR imaging is non-invasive and non-ionizing. Any plane for sectioning the heart can be chosen (5). Spatial resolution is just as good as in angiocardiography and echo/Doppler-cardiography. There is no interference from bone- or lung tissue. Apart from excellent anatomic information of the heart, MRI simultaneously delineates bronchial and abdominal anatomy (2, 3, 4), which is of great importance when evaluating complex heart disease as for instance in asplenia- and polysplenia syndromes and other situs anomalies. However, MRI averages information obtained from many consecutive heart beats. Therefore, cardiac rhythm has to be regular and the patient has to lie still. In young children sedation is necessary. The acquisition time for a complete study is from 3/4 to 1½ hours. During this time the patient is out of reach for close supervision by the attending physician. Children on artificial ventilation or with a cardiac pacemaker cannot be studied with MRI. Functional parameters can be derived from MRI: end-systolic and end-diastolic volumes (6), ejection fraction (7), cardiac output, wall motion and wall thickness. With cine-MRI jets from stenotic valves, ventricular septal defects etc. can be visualized as well as the regurgitant blood stream from valvular incompetence. The MRI equipment of course is expensive and requires highly trained personnel.

From the above considerations it seems that MRI lends itself well for the study of complex heart disease, especially in children with situs anomalies; furthermore for the evaluation of the truncus pulmonalis and the proximal pulmonary arteries and of the aorta in its entire course from heart to diaphragm. MRI is, generally speaking, not a suitable technique for the investigation of critically ill infants requiring ventilatory support. Good results can be expected in postoperative patients, especially after arterial switch operation and in those with conduit-operations like the Fontan-, Rastelli-, Senning-, and Mustard operation.

REFERENCES

1. Pohost G and Canby RC.
   Nuclear magnetic resonance imaging: current applications and future prospects.
   Circulation 75: 88-95, 1987.

2. Dinsmore RE, Wismer GL, Levine RA, Okada RD, Brady TJ.
   Magnetic resonance imaging of the heart: positioning and gradient angle selection for optimal imaging planes.
   Amer J Roentgenol 143: 1135-1142, 1984.

3. Guit GL, Bluemm RG, Rohmer J, Wenink AC, Chin JG, Doornbos J, Van Voorthuisen AE.
   Levotransposition of the aorta: identification of segmental cardiac anatomy using MR imaging.
   Radiology 161: 673-679, 1986.

4. Fletcher BD, Jacobstein MD, Nelson AD, Rimmelschneider TA, Alfidi RJ.
   Gated magnetic resonance imaging of congenital cardiac malformations.
   Radiology 150: 137-140, 1984.

5. Didier D, Higgins CB, Fisher MR, Osaki L, Silverman NH, Cheitlin MD.
   Congenital heart disease: gated MR imaging in 72 patients.
   Radiology 158: 227-235, 1986.

6. Kaul S, Wismer GL, Brady TJ, Johnston DL, Weyman AE, Okada RD, Dinsmore RE.
   Measurement of normal left heart dimensions using optimally oriented MR images.
   Amer J Roentgenol 146: 75-79, 1986.

7. Stratemeier EJ, Thompson R, Brady TJ, Miller SW, Saini S, Wismer GL, Okada RD, Dinsmore RE.
   Ejection fraction determination by MR imaging: comparison with left ventricular angiography.
   Radiology 158: 775-777, 1986.

HIGH SPEED IMAGING OF THE HEART

MICHAEL T. McNAMARA

Magnetic resonance (MR) imaging has thus far demonstrated enormous capability for visualization of the normal and pathologic heart (1 - 9). MR has accurately defined normal cardiac anatomy (1), congenital cardiac abnormalities (2), acute myocardial infarction (3), chronic myocardial infarction (4), myocardial ischemia (5), cardiac and paracardiac masses (6), pericardial anatomy and pathology (7), and diseases of the aorta (8). Due to cardiac motion however, it is necessary to gate the image acquisition sequences to the electrocardiographic cycle in order to produce sufficient resolution of the heart (9). Such a technique utilizes standard spin echo pulse sequences and requires between 4-10 minutes for a multisection acquisition. Rapidly flowing blood is characterized by low to absent signal intensity due to spin-phase cancellation effect and due to time-of-flight bulk motion effects.

Recently there have been significant efforts to diminish the MR examination time in order to improve the clinical efficiency of the study. to decrease patient discomfort due to prolonged periods of remaining motionless, and to minimize the image-degrading effects of involuntary physiologic motion. By far the most exciting technique for "fast-scanning" has been the gradient reversal echo, also known as the fast-field-echo (10). This technique has resulted in the ability to acquire dynamic changes of the heart (11) and short breadhold images of the abdomen that are essentially free of respiratory motion artifact (12).

PRINCIPLES

Conventional spin echo images are reconstructed by acquiring a multitude of projections, typically about 128 to 256 per image, each with an identical setting of a readout gradient during which the sequence is sampled. Each projection is differentiated from one another by a phase difference which is produced by advancing the phase encoding gradient. With the spin echo technique each projection is produced by a 90-degree pulse for generation of transverse magnetization, followed by a 180-degree pulse for induction of the spin echo. The total time, T exam, that is required for image acquisition is related to the number of projections, Np, the pulse sequence repetition time, TR, and the number of excitations, N ex, by:

$$T_{exam} = N_p \cdot TR \cdot N_{ex}$$

Image acquisition times may therefore be reduced by decreasing the number

134

of projections and/or the number of exitations, at the expense of reducing image resolution and/or signal-to-noise, respectively. However, if one attempts to reduce the third parameter in the equation, TR, the systems begins to become saturated and the MR signal becomes gradually weaker. The solution to this problem is to utilize flip angles which are less than 90 degrees, which allows the achievement of a steady state in which most of the magnetization remain longitudinal at all times (as opposed the spin echo in which the initial 90-degrees pulse initially places all magnetization in the transverse plane), allowing a proportionately larger gain in transverse magnetization. This technique allows the reduction of TR from hundreds of milliseconds down to the order of tens of milliseconds, thereby shortening the MR examination time.

In order to prevent the longitudinal magnetization from being driven to zero, an additional modification must be made to replace the 180-degree refocusing pulse which characterizes the spin echo. This is accomplished by the gradient reversal echo (Figure 1). To initiate the gradient echo, a negative gradient is applied in the readout direction to produce dephasing of the affected volume of spins. This is followed immediately by a positive gradient to produce the rephasing phenomenon. At our institution in Monaco, we employ a version of this technique which is known as GRASS: Gradient Recalled Echo in the Steady State (Figure 2) (General Electric Signa, Milwaukee, WI).

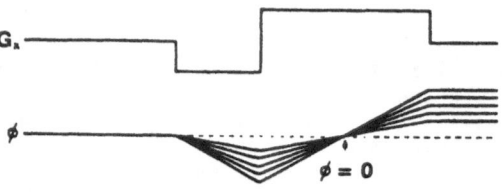

Figure 1. Principle of gradient echo.

During the period of the dephasing lobe of the
readout gradient, the spins lose phase which
they gain back after sign reversal of the
readout gradient. Note that all spins are
back in phase at the center of the
readout gradient. (From FE Werhli,
Introduction to Fast-Scan Magnetic
Resonance. General Electric Company, Medical
Systems Group, Milwaukee, WI. Reproduced with
permission).

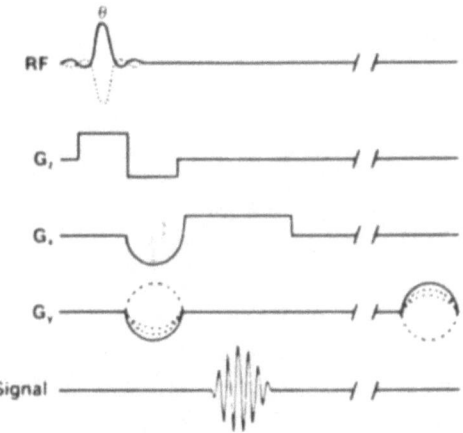

Figure 2. GRASS pulse sequence. The principal
distinguishing features of the GRASS sequence are :

1. The gradient echo caused by sign inversion of the
readout gradient.
2. A rephasing gradient applied at the end of the
sequence to compensate for the view-to-view phase
change induced by the phase encoding gradient.
(From FW Wehrli, Introduction to Fast-Scan Magnetic
Resonance. General Electric Company, Medical Systems
Group, Milwaukee, WI. Reproduced with permission).

VASCULAR EFFECTS OF GRASS

Standard spin echo images typically depict rapidly flowing blood as a
low signal intensity region within the cardiac chambers and vascular lamina. Blood flow may also be characterized by high intensity due to various physical phenomena, such as even echo rephasing (13), flow-related
enhancement on entrance slices (14), and slow or turbulent blood flow
(3,4,15). The GRASS sequence, however provides enhancement for both arteries and veins regardless of position and often regardless of velocity
(Figure 3). This signal enhancement results from the inflow of unsaturated, that is fully relaxed, spins betweens radiofrequency excitations.
GRASS utilizes sequential data acquisition and thus, previously saturated
spins may never enter the imaging volume. At a TR of 21 msec, complete
washout of saturated spins occurs at a flow velocity of 23cm/second (16).
Additionally, since gradient refocusing is not slice selective, moving
spins will be detected even if they are execited within the imaging slice
and then flow out of the slice plane.

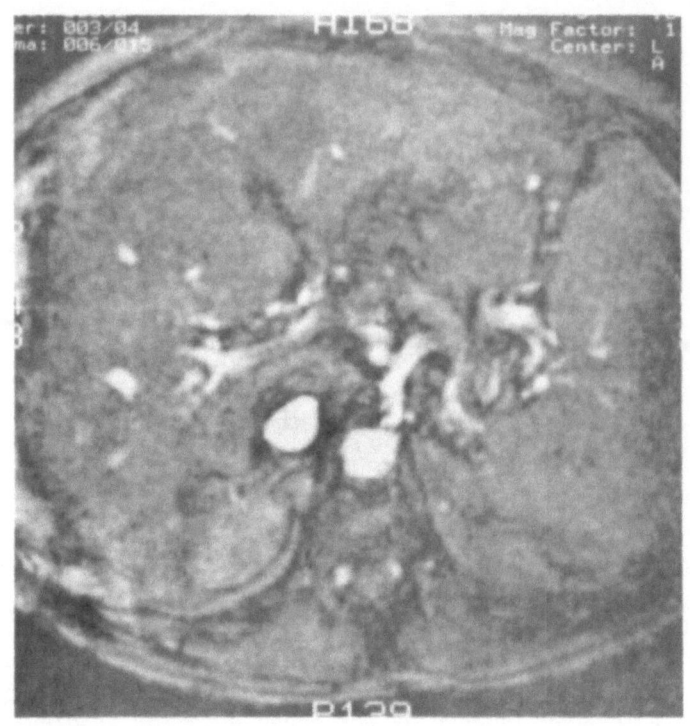

Figure 3. Transverse GRASS image
(TR = 21 msec, TE = 12 msec,
flip angle = 30 degrees) of the abdomen.
Note that the blood within the inferior vena cava,
aorta, and hepatic and splenic vessels are
characterized by high signal intensity.

Due to a net accumulation of phase shift of moving spins at the end of a gradient pulse, there is a tendency for spatial displacement of the intravascular signal.
This is particularly true for flow that is perpendicular to the plane of section. This may be significantly reduced or eliminated by applying a correction gradient which results in equal phase for both flowing and stationary spins (17). This correction gradient may also be applied in the

phase encoding and readout directions.

Initial studies with a fluid-filled flow phantom indicate that signal intensity increases monotonically with increasing flow rate, reaching an asymptote that is independant of TR (18). While the signal intensity from flowing fluid was stable across a range of TR values at a flip angle of 90 degrees, signal from stationary fluid decreased with decreasing TR. Variation of the flip angle demonstrated that signal from flowing fluid increased with increasing flip angle, reaching a peak value at 90 degrees. In contrast, the signal from stationary fluid increased to a maximum value at 40 degrees; above 40 degrees there was a decrease in intensity with increasing flip angle. In summary both TR and flip angle affect vascular contrast. At high flow rates, vascular contrast increases with increasing flip angle because of the increase in signal which characterizes flowing spins and also because of the decrease in signal from stationary spins.

RAPID DYNAMIC MR IMAGING OF THE HEART.

The GRASS MR examination may be gated to the electrocardiographic cycle to produce dynamic images of the heart (Figure 4).

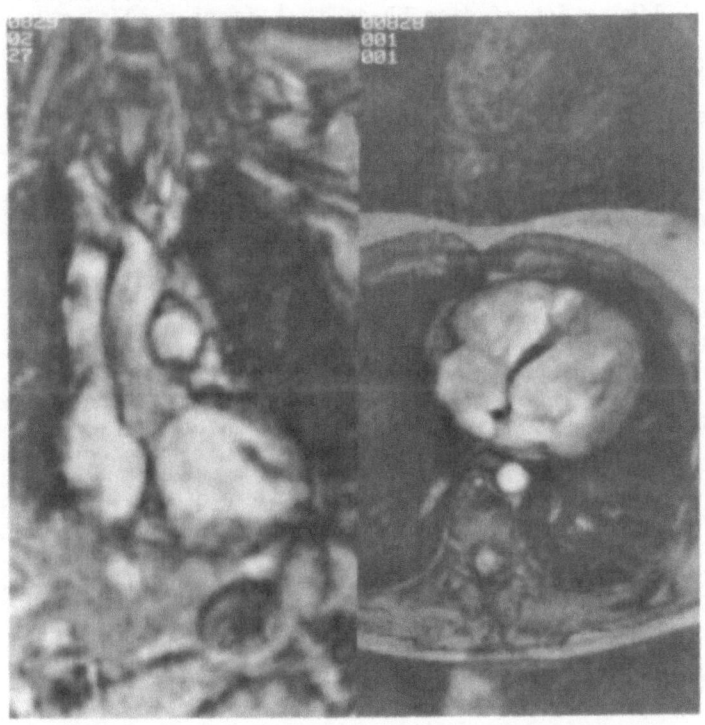

Figure 4. Coronal (left) and transverse (right)
GRASS images of the heart (TR = 21 msec,
TE = 12 msec, flip angle = 30 degrees)
of a normal volunteer. The intracardiac and
intravascular blood flow is hyperintense.
compared to the myocardium and vascular walls.
The mitral value is well visualized.

In our MR system, this is known as CINESCAN. CINESCAN involves a conti-
nuous acquisition of gradient echo MR data utilizing a TR of 21 msec, and
echo delay time of 12 msec, and limited flip angles, generally about 30
degrees. The cine MR exam is gated to the patient's heart rate and the
phase encoding gradient is advanced with each R-wave trigger. Thus, in the
time required for 128 or 256 heart beats, images with a resolution of
either 128 x 256 or 256 x 256, respectively, may be acquired. Up to four
slices may be obtained with each acquisition with a slice thickness of 5
or 10 millimeters, and therefore the entire heart may be studied in less
than 30 minutes. Images may be reconstructed with a temporal resolution of
up to 32 intervals per cardiac cycle.

The quality of the CINESCAN image depends upon the regularity of the
patient's heart rate and is inversely proportional to the standard deviation of the heart rate (19). Image quality can be objectively assessed by
the standard deviation of the number of triggers per image. Images are
also degraded by diaphragmatic motion at the cardiac apex which produces
artifacts in the phase encoding direction. The use of a surface-coil reduces these artifacts and improves the signal-to-noise-ratio. Gradient
echo fast images are more sensitive to susceptibility changes and metallic
artifacts from vascular clips or metallic sutures will degrade image quality. A final limitation of cine MR is that image quality may be degraded
in patients with atrial fibrillation; diagnostically useful images may
still be obtained with these patients, however.

A comparison of cine MR gradient echo studies using varying flip angles
between 22.5 degrees and 90 degrees demonstrated that intravascular blood
was more intense with greater flip angles (19). Intraventricular cardiac
blood however was less intense at higher flip angles, probably related to
turbulence and in-plane flow. Therefore, contrast between the myocardium
and the intracavitary blood was superior at low flip angles.

NORMAL CARDIAC ANATOMY AND CARDIAC PATHOLOGY

NORMAL SUBJECTS. Myocardial wall thickening is readily visualized with
CINESCAN during systole and in normal subjects (11). Right and left
ventricular stroke volumes can be obtained by subtraction of end-diastolic
and end-systolic volumes and have been shown to be nearly identical using
this MR technique. Although intracardiac blood is very intense due to
inflow of unsaturated spins, a small region of signal loss may be seen in
the right atrium in normal subjects, immediately posterior the tricuspid
valve, apparently due to reversal of blood flow in the tricuspid valve
cone with valve closure. A small signal loss may also be seen in early
diastole within the left ventricle close to the mitral valve and on the
ventricular aspects of the atrioventricular valve leaflets during diastole. Cine MR radily demonstrates motion of the cardiac valves.

MYOCARDIAL ISCHEMIA. Areas of previous myocardial infarction are characterized by regions of absent or decreased systolic wall thickening.
Some patients may demonstrate passive systolic inward wall motion without
normal thickening. Cine MR enables estimation of diastolic wall thinning
and aneurysms with chronic myocardial infarcts. Since the cine display
allows visual assessment of cardiac function as indicated by wall motion
and wall thickening, this technique may be more accurate for determination
of infarct size than two-dimensional echocardiography. Mural thrombus is

also readily visualized due to a low signal intensity which is strongly contrasted with the intracavitary blood.

VALVULAR DISEASE. In patients with cardiac valvular regurgitation cine MR depicts the regurgitant jet of flow as a region of low signal intensity which extends from the incompetent valve into the adjacent cardiac chamber. In cases of tricuspid and mitral regurgitation the low intensity jet is noted to be pansystolic with more extensive involvement of the early systolic signal loss noted in normal volunteers. The morphologic abnormalities in tricuspid and mitral prolapse are also identified by cine MR.

In aortic incompetance, cine MR displays a pansystolic low intensity jet which begins at the level of the valve and extends through several levels to the lateral and inferior walls of the left ventricle. Comparison of left and right ventricular stroke volumes reveals a discrepancy from the normally equivalent values.

In aortic stenosis cine MR shows the low intensity jet of flow through the aortic cusps with sudden appearance of low intensity within the left ventricular outflow tract.

Since turbulent flow is known to occur in regions of valvular regurgitation and/or stenosis, it is probable that this mechanism is at least partially responsible for the low intensity jet that is seen with these lesions.

PERICARDIAL DISEASE. Cine MR depicts pericardial effusion as high signal intensity, which may be useful because differentiation between pericardial effusion and pericardial calcification may be difficult using conventional gated MR as they may both be characterized by low signal intensity.

INTRACARDIAC SHUNTS. In patients with intracardiac shunts cine gradient echo MR studies demonstrate shunted blood as a fan-shaped region of low signal intensity which extends from the abnormal communication.

SUMMARY

Gradient reversal echoes may be utilized with ECG-gating to noninvasively provide dynamic images of the cardiovascular system. Preliminary results indicate that this technique may be valuable for assessment of cardiac pathology and for providing functional as well as morphologic information about the heart.

140

REFERENCES

1. Higgins CB, Lanzer P, Stark D, et al. Assessment of cardiac anatomy using nuclear magnetic resonance imaging. J Am Coll Cardiol 1985; 5: 77s-81s.

2. Didier D, Higgins CB, Fisher M, Osaki L, Silverman NH, Cheitlin MD. Congenital heart disease: gated MR imaging in 72 patients. Radiology 1986; 158: 227-235.

3. McNamara MT, Higgins CB, Schechtmann N, et al. Detection and characterization of acute myocardial infarction in man with the use of gated magnetic resonance. Circulation 1985; 71: 717-724.

4. McNamara MT, Higgins CB. Magnetic resonance imaging of chronic myocardial infarcts in man. AJR 1986; 146: 315-320.

5. McNamara MT, Higgins CB, Ehman RL. Revel D, Sievers R, Brasch RC. Acute myocardial ischemia: magnetic resonance contrast enhancement with gadolinium - DTPA. Radiology 1984; 153: 157-163.

6. Amparo EG, Higgins CB, Farmer D, Gamsu G, McNamara MT. Gated MRI of cardiac and paracardiac masses: initial experience. AJR 1984; 143: 1151-1156.

7. Stark DD, Higgins CB, Lanzer P, et al. Magnetic resonance imaging of the pericardium: normal and pathologic findings. Radiology 1984; 150: 469-474.

8. Amparo EG, Higgins CB, Shafton EP. Demonstration of coarctation of the aorta by magnetic resonance imaging. AJR 1984; 143: 1192-1194.

9. Lanzer P, Barta C, Botvinick EH, Wiesendanger HUD, Modin G, Higgins CB. ECG-synchronized cardiac MR imaging; method and evaluation. Radiology 1985; 155: 681-686.

10. Haase A, Matthaei D, Hanicke W, Merboldt KD. FLASH imaging: rapid NMR imaging using low flip-angle-pulses. J Magnetic Resonance 1986; 67: 258-266.

11. Sechtem V, Pflugfelder PW, White RD, et al. Cine MR imaging: potential for the evaluation of cardiovascular function. AJR 1987; 148: 239-246.

12. Edelman RR, Hahn PF, Boxton R, Wittenberg J, Ferrucci JT, Brady TJ. Rapid magnetic resonance imaging with suspended respiration: initial clinical application in the abdomen. Radiology 1986; 161: 125-132.

13. Bradley LG, Waluch V. MR even echo rephasing in slow laminar flow. J Comput Assist Tomogr 1984; 8: 594-598.

14. Valk PE, Hale JD, Crooks LE, et al. MRI of blood flow: correlation of image appearance with spin echo phase shift and signal intensity. AJR 1986; 146: 931-939.

15. Von Schultess GK, Fisher M, Crook LE, Higgins CB. Gated MR imaging of

the heart: intracardiac signals in patients and healthy subjects. Radiology 1985; 156: 125-132.

16. Schmalbrock P, Cornhill JF, Hunter WW, Stiving S. Quantitative flow measurement using gradient recalled acquisition into the steady (GRASS). Presented at the annual meeting of the Society of Magnetic Resonance in Medicine, Montreal, Canada, August, 1986.

17. Glover GH. Flow artifacts in MRI. Theory and reduction by gradient moment nulling. General Electric Medical Systems Applied Science Laboratory Technical Report, 1985.

18. Fram E, Hedlund L, Dimick R, Glover G, Herfkens R. Parameters determining the signal of flowing fluid in gradient refocused imaging: flow velocity, TR, and flip angle. Presented at the annual meeting of the Society of Magnetic Resonance in Medicine, Montreal, Canada, August, 1986.

19. Utz J, Herfkens R, Glover G, et al. Rapid dynamic NMR imaging of the heart. Presented at the annual meeting of the Society of Magnetic Resonance in Medicine, Montreal, Canada, 1986.

MRI IN ACQUIRED HEART DISEASE

A. DE ROOS, S. POSTEMA, X.H. KRAUSS, A.E. VAN VOORTHUISEN

INTRODUCTION

Magnetic Resonance Imaging (MRI) is a very useful imaging modality to demonstrate normal and abnormal anatomy of the heart and great vessels. The high velocity of protons in rapid flowing blood causes only little or no signal, providing natural contrast between the cardiac wall and flowing blood. Contrary to X-ray techniques no intravenous injection of contrast agents is necessary to define the cardiac chambers and vascular structures.

Besides morphologic information, tissue characterization is possible by MR, demonstrating alterations in T 1 and T 2 relaxation times. In acute myocardial infarction an increase in relaxaton times correlates with an increase in the water content of myocardial tissue. Rejection of cardiac transplants is also associated with a change in water content of myocardial tissue, therefore MRI may become a sensitive modality to detect rejection after cardiac transplantation (1). Our early results indicate that it is possible to detect rejection of cardiac transplants in humans by demonstration of significantly prolonged relaxation times.

Rapid imaging techniques are now available to study dynamic flow patterns, valvular regurgitation, and cardiac wall motion. To study the dynamic behaviour of flow and motion the images are displayed in a cine mode (2). Furthermore knowledge of human heart metabolism is expanded by characterization of changes in the 31 P NMR-spectrum from the infarcted myocardium (Fig. 1).

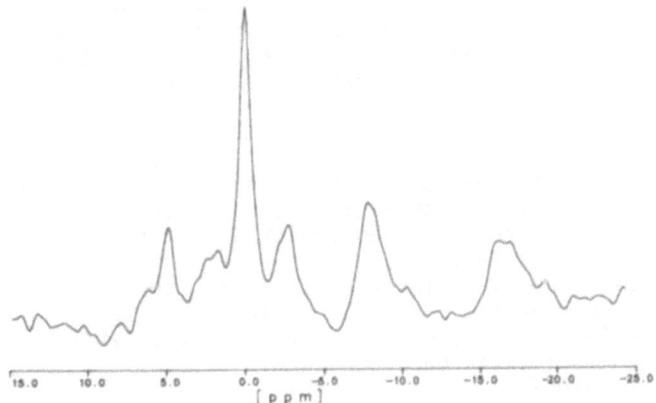

FIGURE 1   In vivo spectroscopy of the human heart. This spectrum was obtained from a normal volunteer by a volume-selective technique. **Note** excellent signal-to-noise ratio. Inorganic phosphate and ATP-peaks are clearly visualized (Philips Gyroscan 1.5 Tesla).

Myocardial infarction

MRI can detect and localize myocardial infarction by demonstrating local wall thinning, increased signal intensity in the infarcted myocardium, and increased signal intensity in the ventricular cavity (3). The thinning of the myocardium is explained by absence of normal systolic thickening of the myocardium in the area of infarction. Increased myocardial wall signal in the infarcted region on spin-echo pulse sequences is due to prolongation of relaxation times (T 1 and T 2). Prolongation of T 1 and T 2 relaxation times in the infarcted myocardium is consistent with myocardial edema. T 2 prolongation appears to predominate and therefore an increased myocardial signal is best appreciated on images with long echo times. We compared the results of thallium imaging and ECG-gated spin-echo MRI to evaluate the potential of both techniques (4).

MATERIAL AND METHODS

Nineteen patients with documented acute myocardial infarction underwent ECG-gated MRI studies of the heart 3-18 days after the diagnosis of infarction had been confirmed. Seventeen patients underwent also Thallium-201 scintigraphy. MRI studies were performed with a 0.5 Tesla superconductive Gyroscan, according to a standard imaging protocol (Table I).

Thallium-201 scintigraphy was performed after intravenous administration of 74MBq (2MCi) TL-201 chloride. Images were obtained immediately following maximum exercise in anterior and oblique projections.

Both MRI and Thallium-scintigraphy were scored by different observers. When both studies assigned the same area as abnormal, this was scored as "correct", when all abnormal areas with MRI were outside the area of decreased uptake at scintigraphy "incorrect" was scored. When one study did not show any abnormality "no findings" were indicated.

RESULTS

The findings of MRI, Thallium scintigraphy, and a comparison between MRI and scintigraphy are summarized in Tables 2-4. MRI detected abnormalities consistent with myocardial infarction in 16/19 patient (84%). Scintigraphy demonstrated perfusion defects consistent with infarction in 15/17 patients (88%).

DISCUSSION

The results of this study demonstrate that MRI can detect and localize acute myocardial infarction with a high accuracy as compared to Thallium scintigraphy. Furthermore, MRI can depict anatomic abnormalities complicating myocardial infarction.

Prolongation of T1 and T2 relaxation times in the infarcted zone are consistent with myocardial edema. T2 prolongation appears to predominate and therefore an increased myocardial signal is best appreciated on images with long echo times (multi-echo technique).

Slowly moving blood in the akinetic infarcted region demonstrates increased intraventricular signal due to rephasing phenomena at even echoes. However, subendocardial increased signal intensity can be difficult to differentiate from flow-related enhancement. Other problems in diagnosing myocardial infarction by MRI is the occurence of an increased myocardial signal intensity, flow-related intraventricular enhancement, and myocardial wall thinning in asymptomatic volunteers. Therefore, application of paramagnetic contrast agents can be useful to enhance contrast between normal and pathological tissue (Fig. 2).

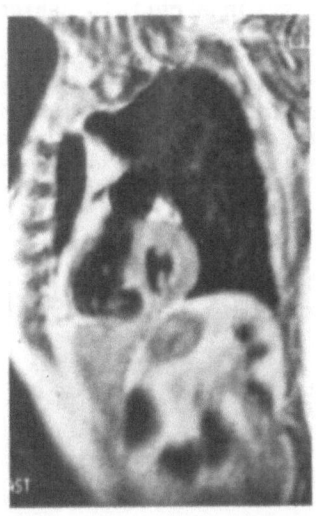 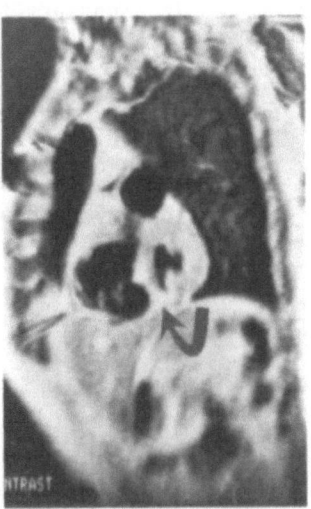

FIGURE 2A Short axis view of left ventricle in patient with recent myocardial infarction with extension into the interventricular
septum. **Note** local thinning of the septum.

2B After intravenous injection of Gadolinium the infarcted area is
clearly demonstrated as an area of high signal intensity (arrow). **Note** small enhancing lesion in the liver.

Gadolinium-DTPA is a clinical useful paramagnetic contrast agent without
adverse reactions. This contrast agent produces local alterations in the
magnetic environment that enhance MR relaxation of protons. Gadolinium
produces significant shortening of T 1 relaxation time of irreversibly
damaged myocardium, resulting in increased signal intensity of the infarct
relative to normal myocardium (5). Both shortening of T 1 relaxation time
and prolongation of T 2 relaxation time will increase MR signal intensity.
The longitudinal (T 1) and transverse (T 2) relaxation times are both
decreased by Gadolinium. In the usual dose of 0.1 mmol per kg body weight
Gadolinium will increase the signal intensity of tissues perfused by this
contrast agent, especially with T 1-weighted pulse sequences.
Thus, Gadolinium permits the use of shorter TR/TE pulse sequences, thereby shortening the imaging time and it may obviate time-consuming T 2
weighted pulse sequences. Gadolinium-enhanced MR images with short echo
times demonstrate a higher signal-to-noise ratio and are less sensitive to
respiratory movements when compared to multi-echo techniques. Therefore,
Gadolinium-enhanced cardiac images with short echo times hopefully can
obviate noisy multi-echo sequences, and improve diagnostic accuracy by
differentiation of increased wall signal from intraventricular flow signal, and increased wall signal due to myocardial infarction from increased
signal intensity in asymptomatic wall segments. Our early results indicate
that increased signal intensity in the infarcted area can be demonstrated
5 minutes after injection of Gd-DTPA. Depending on reperfusion there occurs an increased wash-in of Gadolinium into the infarcted area as well as
a decreased wash-out. A longer diffusion time of Gd-DTPA into an area of

necrosis can make it necessary to wait for a certain period to optimize contrast enhancement.

In conclusion, MRI can detect and localize myocardial infarction with a high accuracy. The results are comparable to the results of Thallium scintigraphy. However, there are several pitfalls which make it necessary to improve MR techniques. Early results indicate that application of Gadolinium as a paramagnetic contrast agent can improve diagnostic accuracy. Furthermore, Gadolinium-enhanced MRI has the ability to distinguish reversible and irreversible myocardial injury.

TABLE I
Imaging protocol for detection of
myocardial infarction

1. Coronal scout view
   * ECG-triggering
   * multi-slice
   * slice thickness 10 mm
   * slice factor 1.5
   * TR 60, TE 30

2. Transverse images
   * trigger-delay 200 msec
   * multi-slice
   * slice thickness 10 mm
   * slice factor 1.1
   * 4 measurements

3. "short-axis" images

4. "long-axis" images

5. Multi-echo single slice image
      (selected slice)
   * TE 30-60-90-120

TABLE II
MRI - Results (n = 19)

A. increased wall signal only	4
B. increased flow signal only	1
C. local wall thinning only	1
D. A + B + C	3
E. A + B	3
F. A + C	4
G. B + C	0
H. no abnormality	3

TABLE III
Thallium - Results (n = 17)

A. persistent perfusion defect   15
B. reversible perfusion defect   3
C. A + B   3
D. no abnormality   2

TABLE IV
A comparison between MRI and Thallium
scintigraphy in detection of myocardial
infarction

Score	Number
No findings	5
Correct	11
Incorrect	1

REFERENCES
1. Aherne, T., Tscholakoff, D., Finkbeiner, W., et al. (1986): Magnetic
Resonance Imaging of Cardiac Transplants: the Evaluation of Rejection of
Cardiac Allografts with and without Immunosuppression. Circulation,
74,1:145-156.

2. Van Dijk, P. (1986): Multiphase mode and cine display permit dynamic
flow MR imaging. Diagn Imag; 163-168.

3. Filipchuk, N.G., Peshock, R.M. Malloy, C.R., et al. (1986): Detection
and Localization of Recent Myocardial Infarction by Magnetic Resonance
Imaging. Am J Cardiol; 58.

4. Krauss X.H., De Roos A., Doornbos J., Van der Wall E.E., Van Voorthuisen A.E., Bruschke A.V.G. (1987): Magnetic Resonance Imaging versus Thal-
lium-201 myocardial perfusion studies in patients with a recent myocardial
infarction. Abstract 36th Annual Scientific Session, American College of
Cardiology, New Orleans, Louisiana 1987. J Am Col Cardiol, 9,2 (suppl A):
74A.

5. Rehr, R.B., Peshock, R.M., Malloy, C.R., et al. (1986). Improved In
Vivo Magnetic Resonance Imaging of Acute Myocardial Infarction After
Intravenous Paramagnetic Contrast Agent Administration. Am J Cardiol, 57:
864-868.

MRI OF THE PULMONARY ARTERIES, AORTA AND VENA CAVA:
CONGENITAL AND ACQUIRED ABNORMALITIES

MURRAY MAZER

MRI OF THE CENTRAL PULMONARY ARTERIES

Pathology imaged:
    a) Congenital Anomalies:

Transposition of great vessels	15
Double outlet right ventricle	4
Truncus arteriosus	2
Patent ductus arteriosus	2
Pulmonary stenosis	14
Pulmonary atresia	5
Pulmonary banding	3
Palliative pulmonary artery shunts	6
Permanent pulmonary artery conduits	5
	56

    b) Acquired Diseases:

Fibrosing mediastinitis	2
Pulmonary embolus	2
Pulmonary hypertension	4
Mediastinal masses	18
	26

Methods:
   All patients were imaged in a 0.5 Tesla superconducting magnet (tesla-con, Technicare - Solan, Ohio).
   Infants and toddlers could be accomodated in a head coil (28 cm diameter). Older children and adults were examined in a 55 cm diameter RF coil; gated, multislice acquisitions from 5.0 - 15 mm. slice thickness were obtained.
   Standard spin-echo images were obtained with an echo-internal (TE) of 30 msec. and pulse repetition rate (TR) of 500 msec.
   Sedation for infants and young children utilized intramuscular Demerol and Seconal, 2 mgm/kg.

Congenital Anomalies:
   MRI's chief imaging competitor is usually echocardiography which is less expensive, portable, truly real-time and does not require gating nor is hindered by rhythm disturbances nor presence of adjacent life-support devices.
   Nevertheless, echocardiography usually cannot image the main, right and left central pulmonary arteries as completely as MRI, especially in older children and adults where sternal ossification, thymic atrophy and interposition of substernal lung tissue limits echocardiographic windows of access.
   When pulmonary artery pressures and vascular resistance measurements are not necessary MRI imaging of the central pulmonary arteries is usually superior to echocardiography and can often replace angiography, particularly for followup evaluations of right heart obstructive diseases and postoperative evaluations of temporary or permanent shunts.

150

Acquired Diseases:
   MRI's chief imaging competitor is usually CT which has faster acquisition time, equal or superior spatial resolution, is not limited by pace-
makers, arrhythmias or life-support devices, which can detect calcium and
is more useful for directing biopsy or drainage procedures. Nevertheless,
MRI can have a selected role to better differentiate lymph nodes from
vasculature and the extent of vascular involvement by mediastinal tumor.
Pulmonary arteriography and cavography can often be eliminated.

MAGNETIC RESONANCE IMAGING OF THE THORACIC AORTA

   This discussion will focus on the role of MRI for evaluation of acquired
diseases of the thoracic aorta (aneurysms and dissection) and congential
diseases involving the thoracic aorta (coarctation, congenital arch anomalies, transposition, systemic-pulmonic collateral circulation shunts and
sequestration).

MRI advantages, to be discussed, include:
   1)   Noninvasive
   2)   No contrast
   3)   No ionizing radiation
   4)   Electronic axis rotation permits infinite imaging
                                                    planes
   5)   Evaluation of flow

MRI limitations, to be discussed, include:
   1)   Image degradation from patient motion
   2)   Current difficulty in monitoring and supporting
        the unstable patient
   3)   Inability to image calcium
   4)   Spatial resolution limitation of subtler vascular
        detail
   5)   Limited evaluation of aortic valve function
   6)   No pressure gradients obtained
   7)   Cost

The thoracic aorta is a relatively simple structure. Aside from coronary
arteries, no subtle, hard to detect branches arise from it. Thus, this is
one area where IV DSA has usually met its expectations. The thoracic
aorta and great vessel takeoffs are usually well assessed by simple IV
DSA in the cooperative patient with reasonable cardiac output and who has
no contraindications for the usual contrast volume required by an IV injection site. Coarctation and thoracic aneurysm workups can often be entirely evaluated by an outpatient IV DSA study. One exception has been in
the area of dissecting aortic aneurysm, where the evaluation of an inti-
mal flap and of false lumen detail has been more discouraging and therefore usually requires more traditional intra-arterial studies. However,
MRI evaluation of a limited number of coarctations and thoracic aneurysms
has provided enough diagnostic information to negate DSA studies entirely, particularly since coronal, sagittal and/or oblique projections provide sufficient evaluation of great vessel relationships to the thoracic
aortic disease. MRI may be all that is needed for evaluation of the more
stable type III dissecting aortic aneurysms and for assessing the fate of
the false lumen size and its flow characteristics on followup examinations.

MRI OF THE INFERIOR VENA CAVA

Pathology Imaged:
- a) Congenital anomalies:
  - Left-sided IVC - isolated   2
  -      - associated with asplenia   2
  - Interruption with azygous continuation (polysplenia)   1
  - Anomalous entry into IVC; retroaortic left renal vein $\frac{1}{6}$

- b) Acquired anomalies:
  - Surgical diversions - splenocaval shunt   2
  -      - caval diversion in transposition repair   14
  - Idiopathic thrombosis   2
  - Abdominal aortic aneurysm - compression   2
  - Abdominal aortic dissection - compression   2
  - Paracaval hemangioma - compression   1
  - Hepatic cyst - compression   2
  - Hepatic metastases - compression   1
  - Hepatoma - invasion   1
  - Pancreatic mass - compression   1
  - Adrenocortical carcinoma - compression   4
  - Adrenal metastases (melanoma) - compression   3
  - Phaechromocytoma - compression   2
  - Retroperitoneal testicular carcinoma - compression   1
  - Wilms tumor - invasion   1
  - Renal adenocarcinoma - invasion (6) compression (5) $\frac{11}{52}$

Conclusions:
Superior spatial resolution and familiarity with CT still warrants its use as one of the principle imaging modalities to first evaluate the abdomen.

However, MRI evaluation of the inferior vena cava can assume prime importance when:
- a) There is further need to delineate vascular anatomy (particularly in longitudinal planes) after CT or ultrasound evaluation.
- b) The patient is pregnant.
- c) The patient is allergic to contrast
- d) Severe renal dysfunction negates the use of contrast.
- e) Tissue characterization (tumor vs thrombus) is necessary; tissue biopsy could then be better directed.

The necessity for inferior venacavography can be considerably diminished. Extrinsic compression by a dorsal or ventral mass is usually best appreciated on sagittal imaging, and by medial or lateral masses with coronal imaging. Intracaval disease is best confirmed by both views to avoid volume-averaging false-positive interpretations.

Intraluminal tumor usually has the same signal as adjacent retroperitoneal tumor. An intraluminal filling defect that expands the lumen suggests malignancy.

Isolated blood clots usually have relatively high signal intensity and do not widen the diameter of the involved vein. Chronic thrombosis may have a more diminished signal secondary to fibrotic changes and appreciated only by the presence of a small residual recanalized lumen.

Future MRI evaluation of the inferior vena cava may improve further with more specific flow imaging, faster acquisition techniques and possible selected enhancement with intravenous paramagnetic contrast agents such as Gadolinium-DTPA.

SECTION IV ABDOMINAL IMAGING

MAGNETIC RESONANCE IMAGING OF THE ABDOMEN

G. M. Bydder

INTRODUCTION

Progress in magnetic resonance imaging (MRI) of the central nervous system has been rapid and now this technique has become established as the technique of first choice in a variety of neurological diseases. Developments in MRI of the abdomen have been slower and the role of MRI is much less clear than it is in the nervous system. Nevertheless there have been some significant technical developments over the last year and results in this region have shown a decided improvement.

TECHNICAL DIFFERENCES BETWEEN MRI OF THE BRAIN AND THE ABDOMEN

One of the most obvious differences between imaging of the brain and that of the abdomen is the degree of movement present. While the brain displays slight pulsatile movement and detectable CSF flow, the effects are small compared to the large scale movements accompanying respiration and peristalsis in the abdomen. These latter movements are not as predictable as vascular pulsation and the longer period of respiration makes gating in the conventional sense a long drawn out process. Whilst peristalsis can be controlled for short periods with drugs such as glucagon the long duration of MRI scans frequently makes this drug unsatisfactory.

Whilst fat in the form of triglycerides is only seen within the CNS in a few pathological circumstances, it is ubiquitous both inside and outside the abdomen. This has two consequences. Firstly the anterior abdominal wall fat is the most frequent source of phase encoded artefact and secondly, if a long TE long TR spin-echo approach is used, lesions which have a relatively long T_2 may simulate fat (whose normal T_2 is relatively long) producing a net loss of contrast.

The short T_2 of many abdominal organs (about half that of brain) has further consequences. For example an inversion recovery sequence which has a high T_1 dependence when used for the brain may have only a moderate T_1 dependence when used for the liver (as a result of the much greater T_2 dependence).

The fluid associated with the brain (i.e. CSF) is uniform, essentially static in position and has a low protein content. None of these facts are true of bowel contents. Their T_1 and T_2 values vary, their position changes and their consistency varies from fluid to semi-solid.

All of these features have created problems in MRI of the abdomen, and the relatively slow progress of development of MRI imaging is not altogether surprising. However solutions or partial solutions to some of these problems have evolved over the last year and some of these are outlined below.

DEVELOPMENT OF "CORSET" COILS

The advantages of surface coils in improving signal to noise ratio were first recognised in spectroscopy (1) but have more recently been applied to MRI (2,3). They are most valuable in imaging small superficial structures so that their advantages in displaying the whole abdomen are rather less. Nevertheless improvements have resulted from the use of closely coupled corset coils applied around the patient's abdomen. The so called 'filling factor' or proportion of the coil volume occupied by the patient is increased and this can result in improved image quality. In order to avoid excessive capacitative coupling the conductors are made of copper tubing.

HIGH RESOLUTION (256 X 256) IMAGING

Until quite recently almost all images of the abdomen were based on a 128 matrix i.e. 128 pixels in the phase encoded direction. The frequency encoded direction was 128, 192 or 256. This provided an upper limit to the resolution of abdominal images. Since X-ray computed tomography (CT) is now performed essentially on a 256 x 256 matrix this put MRI at a disadvantage in terms of spatial resolution. One of the first consequences of the use of corset coils has been the fact that 256 pixel phase encoding images can now be obtained with overall resolution of 256 x 256, 256 x 384 or 256 x 512. As a result of the improved signal to noise ratio MRI is no longer at a disadvantage compared to CT in terms of spatial resolution in imaging of the abdomen (Fig. 1).

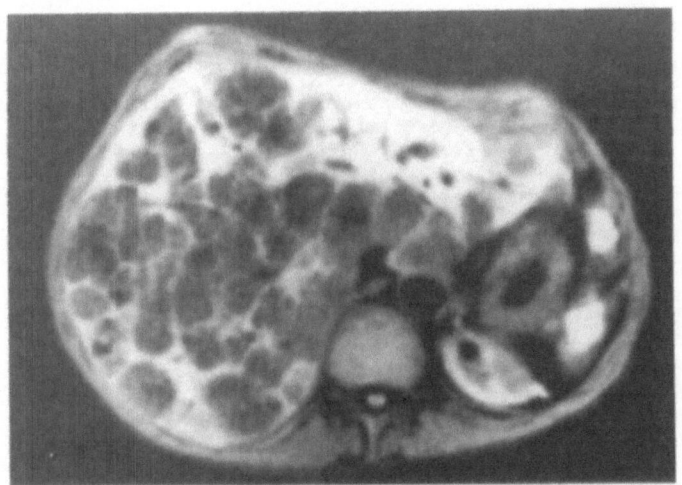

FIGURE 1.   Liver metastases.   High resolution IR1500/500/44 scan (256 x 256 matrix). Metastases are seen at high resolution.

RESPIRATORY ORDERED PHASE ENCODING (ROPE)

While it is possible to use conventional systems of gating to coordinate MRI pulse sequences to the respiratory cycle these produce a considerable prolongation of examination time - typically by a factor of 2 or 3.

An alternative to these gating systems is respiratory ordered phase encoding (ROPE) (4). With this technique the position of the patient's anterior abdominal wall in the vertical or phase encoding direction is monitored. The probability distribution of the position of the patient's abdominal wall is then determined.   During scanning the position of the patient's abdominal wall is monitored and the phase encoding gradient is chosen so that the size of the gradient increases monotomically with the patient's position. This produces a considerable reduction in the 'ghost' artefacts which are frequently seen in the phase encoded direction without incurring a significant time penalty.

USE OF THE SHORT TI INVERSION RECOVERY (STIR) SEQUENCE

Another method of reducing 'ghost' artefacts from the fat of the anterior abdominal wall is the use of an inversion recovery sequence with the TI chosen so that fat is at 'null' point and has zero magnetization at the time of the 90o pulse (5). This sequence also reduces the signal from intra abdominal fat to zero and avoids confusion of lesions with fat. It has the further advantage of making T_1 and T_2 dependent contrast <u>additive</u> so producing high lesion contrast (Fig. 2). In addition, the reduction of the fat signal to zero means that certain types of chemical shift artefact can be controlled.

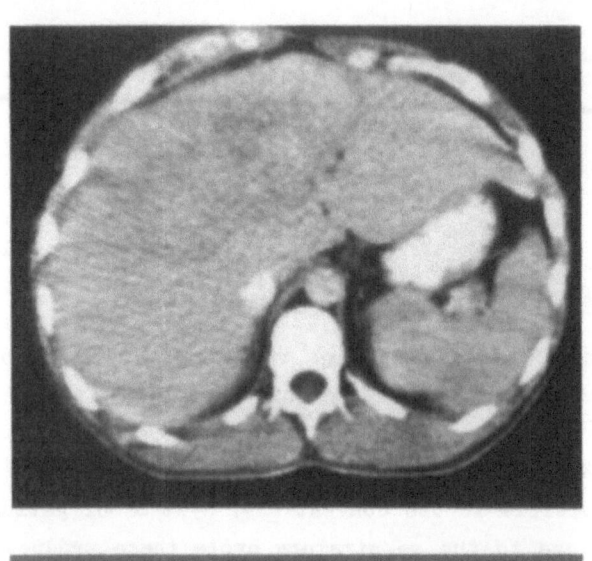

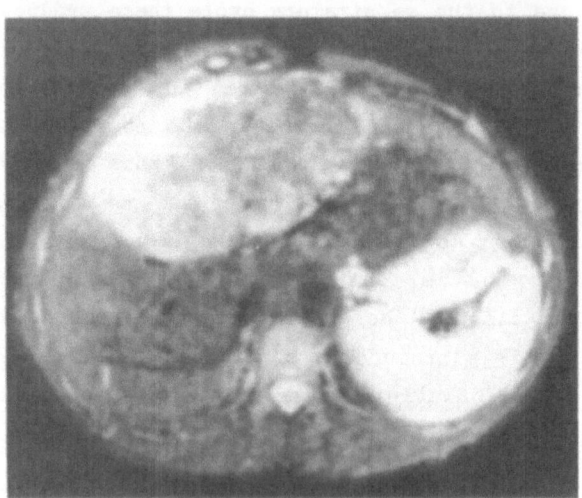

FIGURE 2. Hepatoma: a) contrast enhanced CT and b) IR1500/100/44 scans. The tumour and associated fatty change give a high signal intensity.

sting
highly
hronic
umors.
asound
ole in
refore

e for
h oral
y.
y than
within

ey are

The
study
is to
this

Anot
magnet
Fe_3O_4
limite
concen
signal

THE LI
Init
above
result

Othe
TE seq
(up to

Disadvantages of the sequence include the fact that it is relatively 'noisy' and that the zero signal level may be due to air, calcification, flowing blood or fat. Some of these difficulties may be avoided by pairing the STIR sequence with a short TE short TR spin echo sequence.

USE OF CHEMICAL SHIFT IMAGING TECHNIQUES

The use of phase contrast techniques for separating protons in water from those in lipid was pioneered by Dixon (6) and Seponnen et al (7). These authors described a system of using asymmetrical spin echo sequences in combination with conventional symmetrical spin echo sequences to obtain images reflecting lipid or water content.

The same principle can be used with the partial saturation sequence (8). The most interesting case with this sequence occurs when TE is chosen so that the signals from lipid and water are 180° out of phase and largely cancel out if the proportions of lipid and water are roughly equal. This is of value in the liver where there may be fatty infiltration, in pancreatitis and in diseases involving bone marrow.

CONTRAST AGENTS

The intravenous contrast agent Gadolinium-DTPA has been used in the study of the liver and pancreas over the last year (9). Its major effect is to produce a reduction in T_1 with a smaller reduction in T_2 (although this can be important with higher concentrations of the agent).

Another type of contrast agent - bulk susceptibility agents - based on magnetite have been developed for animal use (10, 11). These consist of Fe_3O_4 particles which are superparamagnetic. They have a relatively limited effect on T_1 but produce a marked decrease in T_2 even in quite low concentrations. These agents may be particularly useful for reducing the signal from bowel contents.

THE LIVER

Initial results in the liver showed promise (12,13) but some of the above mentioned difficulties have proved significant hurdles in achieving results comparable with those of other techniques.

Other significant new developments have included the use of very short TE sequences (e.g. TE = 10 msec) combined with large numbers of averages (up to 18) as performed at the Massachusetts General Hospital. This has resulted in acceptable contrast and adequate control of respiratory artefact. The results of this group (15) and of the Philadelphia group in hemangioma (16) have also been of considerable interest and compare well with those of X-ray CT. Our own results with high resolution STIR sequences have been useful (17). All lesions seen on CT have also been seen with MRI. In addition there have been secondary features adjacent to tumors or in a geographical distribution consistent with fatty infiltration, fibrosis or vascular insufficiency. These features were frequently not seen with CT.

Two other studies have been of interest. The first of these has been the collation and analysis of all published values of T_1 and T_2 for the liver by Bottomley et al (18). The liver is the only organ of the body in which T_1 values of tumors were greater than one standard deviation different from normal values. This provides a theoretical basis for expecting a high level of contrast in clinical practice. The second report of interest has been from the Mallinkrodt group who reported increased sensitivity in detecting metastases using asymmetrical spin echo sequences designed to produce a 180° phase different between lipid and water (19). These authors attributed the increased sensitivity to the presence of subtle and latent fatty infiltration accompanying the metastatic lesions.

THE PANCREAS

The pancreas presents a number of special problems. The existing diagnostic technique for the pancreas are quite specific and highly refined. For example, ERCP is highly sensitive and specific for chronic pancreatitis but of much less value in detecting small endocrine tumors. The converse is true of angiography. CT is more valuable than ultrasound in detecting complications of pancreatitis but probably less valuable in detecting small tumors. The specific role for a new technique is therefore difficult to predict.

Control of the signal from bowel is an important prerequisite for pancreatic imaging and so far this has only been partly achieved with oral iron. Glucogen and gas tablets are also not particularly satisfactory.

Nevertheless it is possible to identify tumors with greater clarity than with CT and it is possible to identify inflammatory change within intraabdominal fat.

Changes may also be seen in pancreatitis (Fig. 3) where they are difficult to visualise with CT.

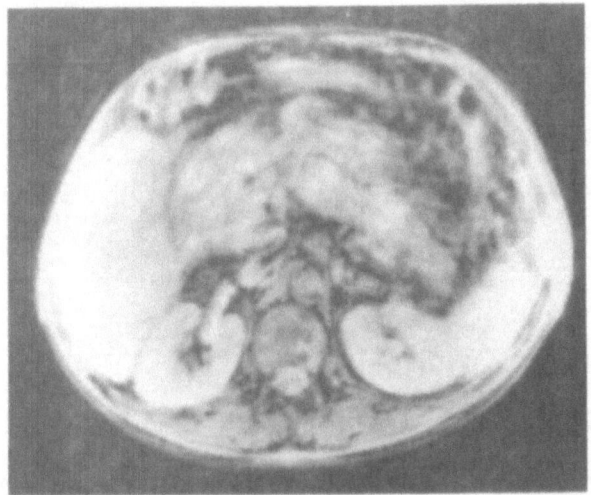

FIGURE 3. Pancreatitis PS500/22 scan. There is a 'cancellation' of the signal from intra-abdominal fat which gives a low signal.

CONCLUSION

Significant progress in MR imaging of the abdomen has been made in the last year but significant problems remain, particularly in relation to the identification of loops of bowel.

There are several new possibilities for coil development although the scope in the abdomen is relatively limited.

Gd-DTPA may be used in association with fast sequences of the steady-state free precession type. Although these sequences are relatively insensitive to disease they may be of much more value following use of Gd-DTPA both in detection of disease and following the uptake and excretion of Gd-DTPA.

Flow measurement techniques have developed over the last year and may have a small role in abdominal disease.

The use of the partial saturation with a reduced flip angle offers the possibility of imaging the abdomen in times of 2-20 sec which are within breath-holding periods (Fig. 4). So far there has been difficulty in developing useful soft tissue contrast and controlling vascular artefacts but this approach may yet prove to be the most useful in screening the abdomen for disease.

162

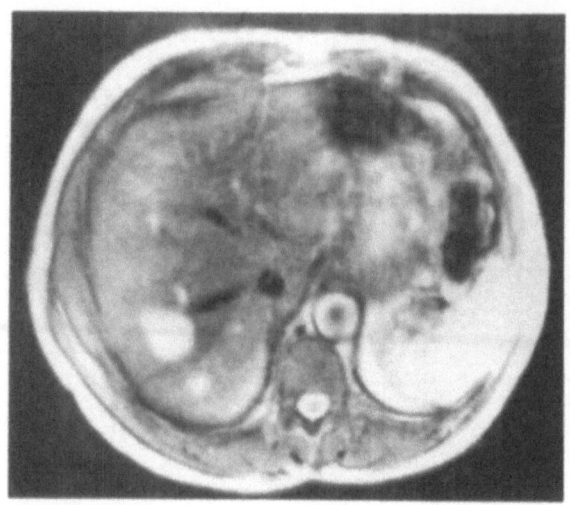

FIGURE 4. Liver metastases PS100/33 image (30° flip angle). Two metastases are seen in the lower right lobe.

REFERENCES

1. Ackerman JH, Grove TH, Wong GG, Gadian DG, Radda GK: Mapping of metabolites in whole animals by ^{31}P NMR using surface coils. Nature 283: 167-170,1980

2. Axel L: Surface coil magnetic resonance imaging. J Comput Assist Tomogr 8: 381-384,1984

3. Bydder GM, Curati WL, Gadian DG, Hall AS, Harman RR, Butson PR, Gilderdale DJ, Young IR: Use of closely coupled receiver coils in MRI: Practical aspects. J Comput Assist Tomogr 9(5): 987-996,1985

4. Bailes DR, Gilderdale DJ, Bydder GM, Collins AG, Firmin DN: Respiratory ordered phase encoding (ROPE): a method for reducing respiratory motion artefact in magnetic resonance imaging. J Comput Assist Tomogr 9(4): 835-838,1985

5. Bydder GM, Young IR: MRI: Clinical use of the inversion recovery sequence. J Comput Assist Tomogr 9(4): 659-675,1985

6. Dixon WT: Simple proton spectroscopic imaging. Radiology 153: 189-194,1984

7. Sepponen RE, Sipponen JT, Tanttu JI: A method for chemical shift imaging: demonstration of bone marrow involvement with proton chemical shift imaging. J Comput Assist Tomogr 8: 585-587,1984

8. Bydder GM, Young IR: Clinical use of the partial saturation and saturation recovery sequences in MR imaging. J Comput Assist Tomogr 9(6): 1020-1032, 1985

9. Carr DH, Graif M, Bydder GM, Niendorf HP, Brown J, Steiner RE, Blumgart LH, Young IR: Gadolinium-DTPA in the assessment of liver tumours by magnetic resonance imaging. Book of Abstracts Society of Magnetic Resonance in Medicine, Fourth Annual Meeting August 19-23, 1985, The Barbican London, UK, Vol 2 pp 1135-1136

10. Mendonca-Dias DH, Bernardo ML, Muller RN, Acuff V, Lauterbur PC: Ferromagnetic particles as contrast agnets for magnetic resonance imaging. Book of Abstracts Society of Magnetic Resonance in Medicine, Fourth Annual Meeting August 19-23, 1985, The Barbican London, UK Vol 2 pp 887-888

11. Olsson M, Persson BRB, Salford LG, Schroder U: Ferromagnetic particles as contrast agent in T_2 NMR imaging. Book of Abstracts Society of Magnetic Resonance in Medicine, Fourth Annual Meeting August 19-23, 1985, The Barbican London, UK, Vol 2 p 889

12. Smith FW, Mallard JR, Reid A, Hutchison JMS: Nuclear magnetic imaging in liver disease. Lancet i: 963-966,1981

13. Doyle FH, Pennock JM, Banks LM, McDonnell MJ, Bydder GM, Steiner RE, Young IR, Clarke GJ, Passmore T, Gilderdale DJ: Nuclear magnetic resonance (NMR) imaging of the liver: initial experience. AJR 138: 193-200,1982

14. Stark DD: MRI of the liver. Teaching Session, Society of Magnetic Resonance in Medicine, Fourth Annual Meeting August 19-23, 1985, The Barbican London, UK.

15. Stark DD, Felder RC, Wittenberg J, Saini S, Butch RJ, White ME, Edelman RR, Mueller PR, Simeone JF, Cohen AM, Brady TJ, Ferruci JF: Magnetic resonance imaging of cavernous haemangioma of the liver: tissue specific characterisation. AJR 145: 213-222,1985

16. Kressel HY, Haggar A, Axel L, Mezrich R, Gefter W: Magnetic resonance imaging of hepatic hemangiomas. Book of Abstracts Society of Magnetic Resonance in Medicine, Fourth Annual Meeting August 19-23, 1985, The Barbican London, UK, Vol 2 p 1164

17. Bydder GM, Steiner RE, Blumgart LH, Khenia S, Young IR: MRI of the liver using short TI inversion recovery sequences. J Comput Assist Tomogr 9(6): 1084-1089,1985

18. Bottomley PA, Hardy CJ, Argersinger RE, Allen GR: Relaxation in pathology: are T_1's and T_2's diagnostic? Book of Abstracts Society of Magnetic Resonance in Medicine, Fourth Annual Meeting August 19-23, 1985, The Barbican London, UK pp 28-29

MRI OF ADRENAL DISEASE

T.H.M. FALKE, A.P VAN SETERS, M.P. SANDLER, M.I. SHAFF

INTRODUCTION

Recent studies advocate Magnetic Resonance Imaging (MRI) of the adrenals as an alternative to more invasive procedures in those cases where CT is equivocal (1-12). MRI shares with Ultrasound (US) a number of advantages over CT, most important of which is the ability to acquire multiplanar images directly without the hazard of ionizing radiation.

In addition MRI generates images with greater inherent tissue contrast than CT, in the absence of streak artefacts from bone or metallic clips. At present the advantages of abdominal MRI are offset by MRI's poorer anatomic resolution which is at least in part consequent on respiratory motion and bowel peristalsis. It is anticipated that the introduction of newer acquisition techniques and tailored surface coils will resolve this problem (10, 13, 14).

NORMAL ADRENALS

The shape of the adrenals on MRI depends on the selected plane and level of sectioning (10). The signal intensity of the normal adrenals is moderate to low depending on the sequence used and is similar to the intensity of the liver. Contrary to CT, enhancement with i.v. contrast material on MRI results in decreased delineation from retroperitoneal fat (Figure 1). MRI is not able to differentiate cortex from medulla either with or without i.v. injection of contrast materials.

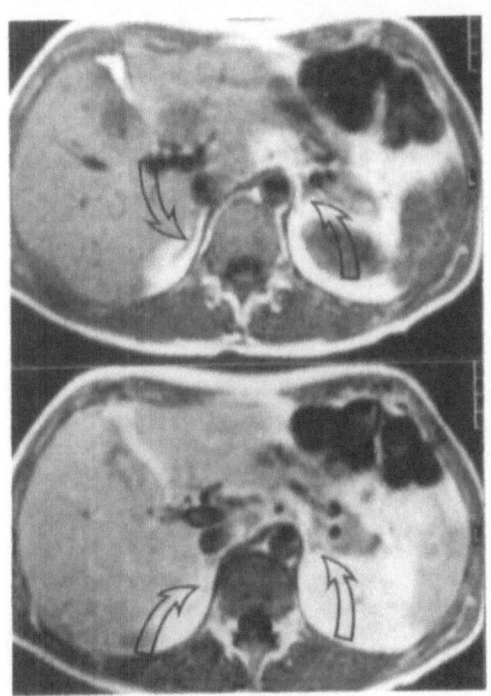

Fig. 1. (A, B).

SE 500/30 before and after 0,1 mmol/kg body weight i.v. GD-DTPA. Normal axial MRI anatomy of the adrenals. After i.v. enhancement with contrast material there is decreased delineation from retroperitoneal fat.

PATHOLOGY OF THE ADRENAL CORTEX
Hyperplasia and adenoma in endocrine disease.
Adrenal hyperplasia is seen on MRI as symmetrical enlargement of the glands with preservation of normal shape, contour, and intensity. Exceptionally in cases of macronodular hyperplasia individual nodules may become large enough to be visualized on MRI and may give rise to problems in differential diagnosis (10).

Adenomas are visualized as small, rounded and well-circumscribed masses. They are usually larger than 2 cm diameter in Cushing's syndrome and usually smaller than 2 cm diameter in primary hyperaldosteronism. On MRI the intensity may be iso- or hyperintense (4, 10, 19) as compared to the liver on T2 weighted sequences. The use of MRI in this patient group awaits further improvement of the resolution of the MR image.

Non-hyperfunctioning adenoma
The significance of nodular adrenocortical changes without evidence of steroid overproduction has long puzzled both pathologists and clinicians and has also become a controversial issue in imaging. As an entity it is considerably more common than functioning tumors, and has an incidence at autopsy ranging from 3% for macronodules to 66% for microscopic nodules (15). Large nodules, with a diameter of 2-3 cm, are reported as incidental findings in 0.6-1% of routine upper abdominal CT studies. The number of and size of nodules tends to increase with age and the presence of hypertension, is presumably due to vascular changes within the adrenal cortex.

They more often occur in combination with renal cell and lung carcinoma. The use of MRI to differentiate non-hyperfunctioning adenomas (nodules)

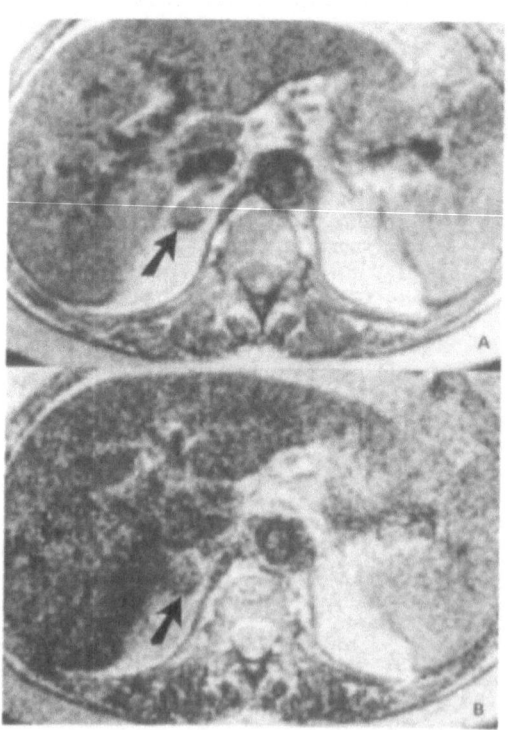

Fig. 2. (A, B).
Non-hyperfunctioning adenoma of the right adrenal gland. **Note** the low signal intensity on T2 weighted sequences.

A: SE 50/2000
B: SE 100/2000.

from other adrenal tumors including metastases has been recently suggested
(1-14). Non-hyperfunctioning nodules usually have a low intensity similar
to the normal liver on T2 weighted sequences (Fig. 2) contrary to most
other tumors which usually demonstrate increased intensity relative to the
liver. However results also demonstrate an area of overlap that occurs due
to non-hyperfunctioning adenomas with high cellularity (20) hemorrhage and
cystic changes (20) and due to metastasis originating from a primary tumor
with a relative low signal intensity, such as tumors from the digestive
tract (1, 10). Although MRI may be of some use in characterizing incidental adrenal masses in individual patients CT or US guided biopsy or CT
follow-up is required if a definitive diagnosis is crucial to patient management.

Carcinoma
    Presenting signs and symptoms of malignant adrenocortical tumors depends
on the nature of steroid overproduction, the size of the tumor and the
presence of metastases as well as the sex and age of the patient.
    When biosynthetic potency is low, patients present with abdominal pain,
palpable mass, metastases, malaise, weight loss and fever, but without
endocrine manifestations.
    The majority of the carcinomas are large enough to be visualized by
conventional radiographic methods such as plain abdominal films or intravenous pyelography. On CT, US and MRI tumors are generally distinguishable
from adenomas by their large size, irregular and lobulated borders and the
occasional presence of infiltration and metastases. Primary carcinomas of
the adrenal cortex usually have an increased signal intensity relative to
that of the liver on SE sequences with a long TR/TE (Fig. 3). Depending on

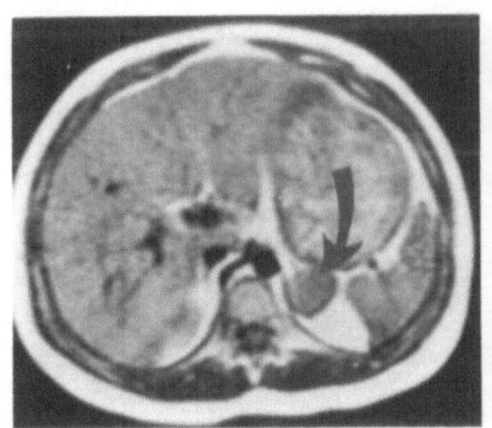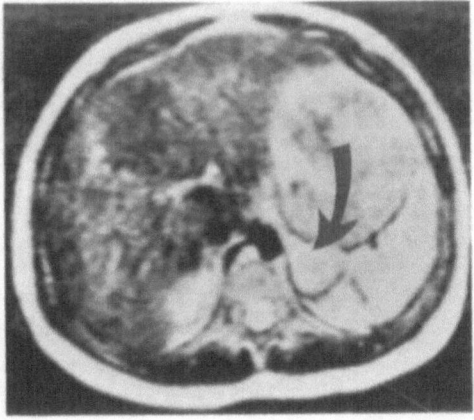

Fig. 3 (A, B).
Child with left adrenocortical carcinoma.
A: SE short TR/TE.
B: SE long TR/TE.

the histologic index ocassionally the signal intensity may be low on all
sequences (10). Sectional imaging techniques are useful to confirm the
diagnosis, to establish tumor extent prior to surgery, to monitor the effect of chemotherapeutic treatment and to detect local recurrence after
surgical treatment. The advantage of optimal plane selection and superior
contrast as compared with CT enables MRI to better evaluate tumor
extent in relation to surrounding structures including major vessels (Fig.
4).

MRI is especially preferred to exclude recurrent tumor in postoperative
patients when metallic clips degrade the CT image (Fig. 5).

Hemorrhagic destruction
Extensive adrenal hemorrhage may occur at any age and under various
circumstances. It is usually associated with severe stress as in surgery,
sepsis, burns, hypotension, trauma and hemorrhagic diatheses. MRI can be
of additional help to CT in establishing the diagnosis when it reveals
high signal intensity in the mass on T1 and T2 weighted sequences (Fig.
6). These findings are probably due to the formation of methamoglobin,
which has paramagnetic properties. Typical characteristics on MRI may be
absent especially in hematomas of less than 48 hrs duration.

In neonates US and MRI are helpful to detect adrenal hemorrhage, differentiate adrenal masses from renal masses and identify simultaneous renal
vein thrombosis without the use of radiation and intravenous contrast
agents or radiopharmaceuticals.

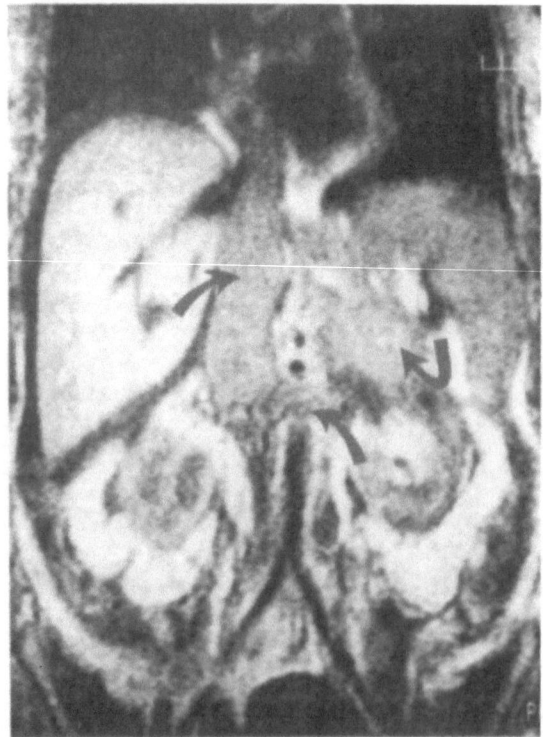

Fig. 4 SE short TR/TE.
Patient with left adrenocortical carcinoma extending into the IVC and
right atrium.

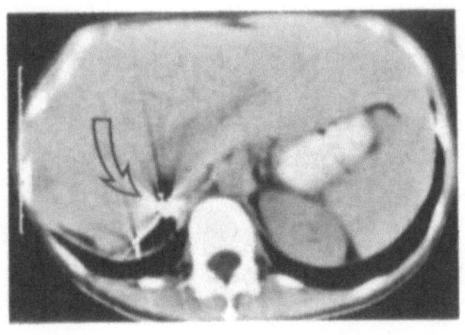

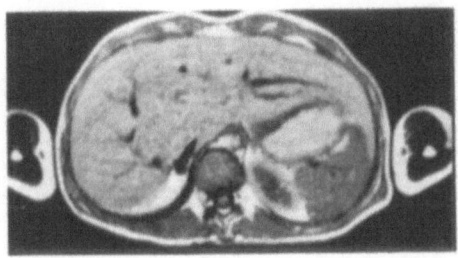

Fig. 5. (A, B). Patient after surgical treatment of right adrenal carci-
noma.
A: CT image is non-diagnostic due to metallic clip artifacts.
B: MRI clearly outlines anatomy. There is no evidence of recurrent tumor.

Adrenal cyst

Cysts may present in any size and in most instances are unilateral. On
MRI an uncomplicated cyst has a negative signal on Inversion Recovery (IR)
sequences and a low signal intensity on spin echo (SE) sequences with a
short time to recovery (TR). On sequences with a long TR/TE the cysts have
a more or less bright signal intensity depending on the protein content.
When hemorrhage or infection occurs in a cyst a very bright signal is observed on short TR sequences (Fig. 7). The appearances of a hemorrhagic or
infected cyst have been described by various authors and the findings on
MRI have proved to be a useful non-invasive way of detecting cyst complications (Fig. 6) and (Fig. 8).

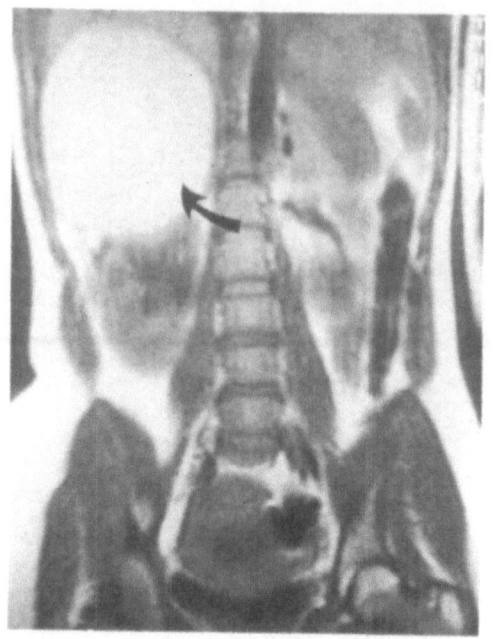

Fig. 6.
Pregnant patients with hemorrhage in a right adrenal cyst. Coronal section
on MR (SE 500/30) demonstrates a high signal intensity lesion consistent
with hemorrhage in a preexisting cyst.

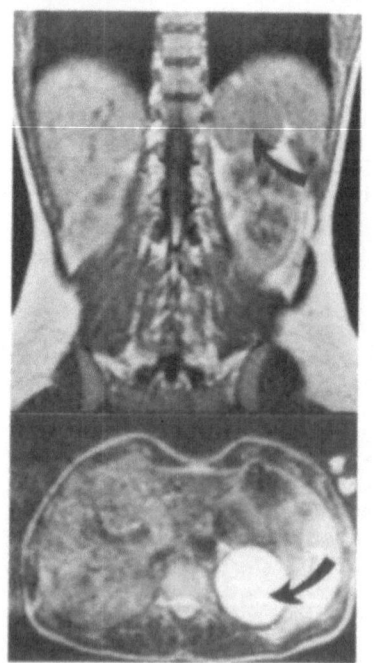

Fig. 7 (A, B).
A: SE short TR/TE
B: SE long TR/TE.

Uncomplicated left adrenal cyst.

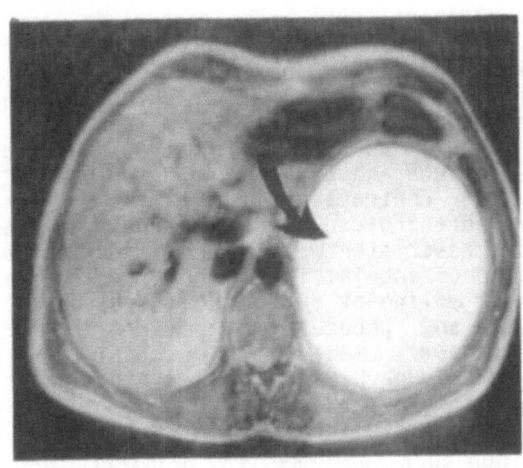

Fig. 8.
SE long TR/Short TE
Infected left adrenal cyst.

Myelolipoma

Adrenal myelolipomas are benign tumors comprising fat and bone marrow elements.

On MRI myelolipomas usually have an increased intensity relative to the liver both on short and long TR SE sequences depending on the amount of fat. They may be inhomogenous or low in intensity depending on the percentage of other tissue components present in the tumor. The absence of a relative increase in signal intensity compared with retroperitoneal fat on long TR/long TE sequences separates myelolipomas with a high fat content from hematomas.

PATHOLOGY OF THE ADRENAL MEDULLA

Pheochromocytoma

Pheochromocytoma occurs in about 0.1% of hypertensive patients. Fifty percent of patients with pheochromocytomas present with paroxysmal hypertensive episodes and fourteen percent of the patients have atypical or absent clinical signs. Patients usually display various elevated patterns of urine and plasma catacholamines and their metabolites although biochemical findings may be absent, especially in the MEN syndrome. Pheochromocytomas originate form chromaffin cell nests along the autonomic ganglia chain or chromaffin bodies such as the adrenal medulla or organ of Zuckerkandl. In adults 90% of the pheochromocytomas are located in one adrenal gland and 10% occur bilaterally. Most ectopic pheochromocytomas are located in the abdomen (9%). Unusual locations include the chest (1%) and urinary bladder (1%). Other localizations such as the heart and kidneys have been described, but are extremely rare. In children and patiens with associated neurocristopathies (MEN, neurofibromatosis) the incidence of bilateral or ectopic localizations is higher.

Pheochromocytomas are considered malignant when they occur in areas outside the normal distribution of chromaffin tissue. Frequent sites of metastases are bone, lymph nodes, lung and liver. In case of malignancy venous involvement into the IVC may occur by direct invasion through the venous wall or by extension along the adrenal veins.

As pheochromocytomas are usually larger than 3 cm in diameter, and located in the adrenals, most of the lesions are detected on CT or MRI. MRI might be performed as initial study over contrast enhanced CT in patients not adequately treated with alpha adrenergic blockades thereby avoiding the small risk of hypertensive crises associated with i.v. injection of contrast materials (17). MRI might be of special interest in more complex cases such as ectopic localizations or malignant dissiminated pheochromocytomas, recurrent pheochromocytoma and pheochromocytomas or medullary hyperplasia associated with MEN II syndrome. Radionuclide scanning with iodine-131 or iodine-123 labelled meta-iodobenzylguanidine synthesized at the University Hospital, Ann Arbor, Michigin, USA is valuable in this group of patients (16). However the results of radionuclide studies have to be confirmed by an imaging technique such as MRI to eliminate both false-positive and false-negative findings and to provide anatomical evaluation prior to surgery. It has been demonstrated that MRI can easily localize and identify pheochromocytomas by their very high signal intensity on T2 weighted sequences (Fig. 9). The combination of optimal plane selection and superior contrast resolution as compared with CT are beneficial to confirm localizations found by nuclear medicine or as alternative when CT is equivocal.

In addition the bright signal intensity on T2 weighted sequences is useful to differentiate pheochromocytomas from adenomas in hypertensive patients when clinical findings are inconclusive.

The use of i.v. contrast material enhancement however is essential to differentiate pheochromocytomas from non-complicated cysts (Fig. 10).

In case of malignant pheochromocytomas MRI is helpful to delineate tumors from surrounding structures including vessels (Fig. 5).

Neuroblastoma and ganglioneuroma

Neuroblastoma is a common tumor in children less than five years old (85%). Prognosis depends on the onset of the disease but is usually poor after the neonatal period. Cyto-differentiation to a more benign ganglionneuroma may occur. All intermediate levels of differentiation between neuroblastoma and ganglioneuroma may be encountered, referred to as ganglioneuroblastoma.

The tumors arise from primordial neural crest cells, and are found in a variety of locations. The adrenal medulla or adjacent retroperitoneum account for 50 to 80% of the tumors. Clinical symptoms may vary and are related to the rapid growth of the neoplasm and its secretory products (norepenephrine, dopa or dopamine) which results in increased urinary levels of their derivates (VMR, HVA and 3-methoxyl-4 hydroxyphenolglycol).

Computed Tomography and Ultrasound have proven to be indispensable tools for diagnosing and following these tumors. Radionuclide studies with the employement of 131-1-MIBG as tracer has attracted much interest, especially with regard to the suggested concomitant therapeutic properties of the isotope.

Recent studies strongly advocate the alternative role of MRI in this group of patients to demonstrate primary and metastatic disease as an aid

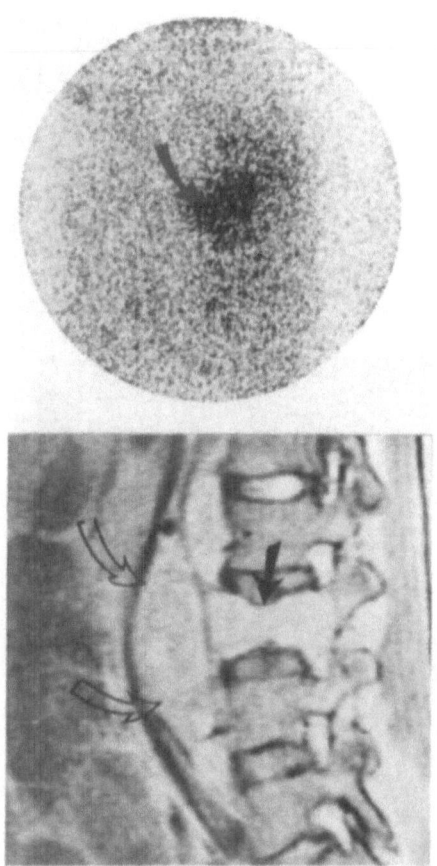

Fig. 9. (A, B)
A: demonstrates uptake of I131-MIGB in the pheochromocytoma, 48 hrs after
injection.
B: Sagittal MRI demonstrating the pheochromocytoma compressing the IVC and
involving the vertebral body. The tumor also encroaches behind the aorta.
SE 45/2000 (case courtesy M.P. Sandler ref. 16 and 20, previously published).

in predicting tumor respectability (5, 8). Particularly the dumbell extension into, or primary location in the epidural space of the spinal canal as well as the relation to major vessels can be non-invasively demonstrated using the advantages of superior contrast and optimal plane
selection. As in most other tumors that arise from neural tissue elements
such as pheochromocytomas and neurofibromas, neuroblastomas have a very
high signal intensity relative to the liver on T2 weighted sequences.

CONCLUSIONS
   Because of limitations in state of the art MRI, as for example the low
anatomical resolution, the major role of MRI at present is complementary
to CT. MRI might be preferred as the initial study when exposure to radiation is considered a relative contraindication, as in children or
pregnant patients; or when reaction to intravenous iodine contrast agents
is anticipated.

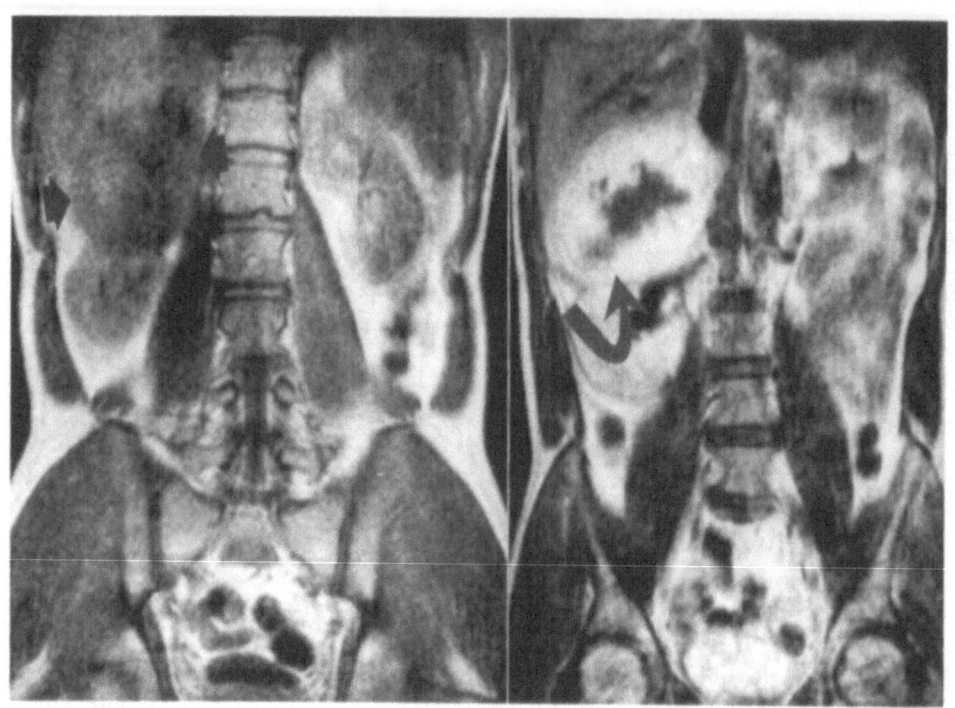

Fig. 10 (A, B).
A: SE short TR/TE before i.v. injection of 0,1 mmol/kg body weight
Gd-DTPA.
B: short TR/TE after i.v. injection of 0,1 mmol/kg body weight Gd-DTPA.
There is periferal enhancement of the pheochromocytoma and increased de-
lineation from the liver (case courtesy dr.med. R.G. Bluemm ref. 20,
previously published).

REFERENCES
1. Reinig JW, Doppman JL, Dwyer AJ, Frank J. MRI of Indeterminate Adrenal Masses. AJR 1986; 147: 493-496.
2. Reinig JW, Doppman JL, Dwyer AJ, Johnson AR, Know RH. Adrenal masses Differentiated by MRI. Radiology 1986; 158: 81-84.
3. Reinig JW, Doppman JL, Dwyer AJ, Johnson AR, Know RH. Distinction between Adrenal Adenomas and Metastases Using MR Imaging. JCAT 1985; 9(5): 898-901.
4. Falke THM, Te Strake L, Shaff MI, Sandler MP, Kulkarni MV, Partain CL, Nieuwenhuijzen Kruseman AC, James AE Jr. MR Imaging of the Adrenals: Correlation with Computed Tomography. JCAT 1986; 10(2): 242-253.
5. Fletcher BD, Kopiwoda SY, Strandjord SE, Nelson AD, Pickering SP. Abdominal Neuroblastoma: Magnetic Resonance Imaging and Tissue Characterization. Radiology 1985; 155: 699-703.
6. Fisher MR, Higgins CB, Andereck W. MR Imaging of an Intrapericardial Pheochromocytoma. JCAT 1985; 9(6): 1103-1105.
7. Fink IF, Reinig JW, Dwyer AJ, Doppman JL, Linehan WM, Keiser HR. MR Imaging of Pheochromocytomas. JCAT 1985; 9(3): 454-458.
8. Cohen MD, Weetman R. Provisor A, McGuire W, McKenn Smith, Carr B, Siddiqui A, Mirkin O, Seo I, Klatte EC. Magnetic Resonance Imaging of Neuroblastomas with a 0.15 T Magnet. AJR 1985143: 1241-1248.
9. Schultz CL, Haaga JR, Fletcher BD, Alfidi RJ, Schultz MA. Magnetic Resonance Imaging of the Adrenal Glands: a Comparison with Computed Tomography. AJR 1984; 143: 1235-1240.
10. Falke THM, Te Strake L, Sandler MP, Shaff MI, Page DL, Bloem JL, Van Seters AP, et al. Magnetic Resonance Imaging of the Adrenal Glands. Radiographics 1987; 7(2): 343-370.
11. Mezrich R, Banner MP, Pollack HM. Magnetic Resonance Imaging of the Adrenal Glands. Urol Radiol 1986; 8(3): 127-138.
12. Schultz CL. CT and MR of the Adrenal Glands. Semin US, CT and MR. 1986; 7(3): 219-233.
13. BLuemm RG, Koops W, Den Boer J, Doornbos J, Van Dijk P. Van der Meulen P, Cuppen J. Fast small flip-angle field echo (FFE) imaging. Textbook Partain (in press).
14. Ferrucci JT. MR imaging of the liver. AJR 1986; 147: 1103-1116.
15. Glazer HS, Weyman PJ, Sagel SS, Levitt RG, McClennan BL. Non-functioning adrenal masses: Incidental discovery on computed tomography. AJR 1982; 139: 81-85.
16. Gross MD, Shapiro B, Sandler MP, Falke THM. Localization of adrenocorticaland sympathomedullary disorders. In: Nuclear Medicine and Correlative Imaging, Williams and Wilkinson, in press.
17. Radin DR, Ralls, PW, Boswell WD Jr, Colletti PM, Lapin SA, Halls JM. Pheochromocytomas: Detection of Unenhanced CT. ARRS 1986; 146: 741-744.
18. Ackery D, Tippet P, Marley A, Weynhove C. Letter to the editor. Lancet 1984; 1: 733.
19. Falke THM, Peetoom JJ, De Roos A. Intravenous extension of adrenocortical carcinoma: MRI evaluation with Gd-DTPA. Radiology 1987; submitted for publication.
20. Falke THM, Shaff MI, Van Seters AP, Sandler MP. Diagnostic Imaging of Adrenal Disease. In: Surgery of the adrenal gland, Scott HW (ed.), Blackwell Scientific Publications, in press.

MAGNETIC RESONANCE IMAGING OF THE BLADDER

Janet E Husband

INTRODUCTION

Despite the introduction of chemotherapy, improvements in surgery and more
sophisticated radiotherapy the overall survival of patients with bladder
cancer has not significantly changed over the past two decades [1,2]. The
two year survival rate for patients with invasive tumours is less than 50%
and the five-year survival figures for superficial tumours not invading
the muscular layers of the bladder wall is approximately 65% [3,4,5].
Apart from the depth of tumour infiltration other factors influencing
prognosis include histological grading and the presence of lymph node
metastases.

Bladder cancer is relatively common accounting for 6% of all male cancers
in the United States and 2% of female cancers. It is estimated that
approximately 11,000 patients die from bladder cancer in the United States
each year [6].

Accurate staging is the key to appropriate management but clinical methods
which include examination under anaesthesia, cystoscopy and biopsy have
been disappointing with errors ranging up to 66% [7,8,9,10]. The main
reason for errors in clinical staging is the difficulty in assessing the
presence and extent of extravesical tumour spread and clinical methods are
thus more accurate for staging superficial than deep infiltrating tumours.

The introduction and rapid development of imaging techniques during recent
years has placed heavy responsibility on the radiologist to provide
accurate staging information. In the assessment of bladder cancer both
ultrasound and CT have proved to be more accurate than clinical staging
alone [11,12,13] but as yet it is too early to make definitive statements
regarding the precise role of magnetic resonance imaging (MRI). Its
potential advantages lie in the ability to obtain images in multiple
planes and the improved contrast sensitivity compared with that of CT.

STAGING CLASSIFICATION

There are two main classifications used throughout the world for staging
bladder cancer. These take into account the depth of bladder invasion and
the presence of metastases in lymph nodes and other sites [14,15,16]. The
International Union Against Cancer (UICC) uses a TNM classification in
which T refers to the extent of the primary tumour, N to lymph node
involvement and M to distant metastases. The Jewett-Strong-Marshall
system corresponds to the TNM classification for staging the primary
tumour but differs with regard to lymph node involvement and distant
metastases.

Clinical staging consists of cystoscopy with biopsy, transurethral
resection, bimanual examination under general anaesthesia as well as other
investigations including excretory urography, chest radiography,
lymphangiography and radionuclide scanning of bone and liver. CT is now
used as an additional staging procedure routinely in many departments and
ultrasound, either employing a transabdominal or transurethral approach,
is also being investigated. MRI is currently being evaluated, in most
studies reported to date the results of this new technique are compared
with those of CT as well as with surgical staging.

PATTERN OF TUMOUR SPREAD

In order to stage tumours accurately it is important that the radiologist
has a detailed knowledge of tumour behaviour and the patterns of spread
which are likely to be seen in advanced disease.

Bladder cancer spreads directly through the muscles of the bladder wall
into the extravesical fat. As disease advances tumour spreads to the
pelvic side wall and into adjacent organs.

Lymph node spread initially occurs in the regional pelvic lymph nodes.
Those first involved include the anterior and lateral paravesical nodes,
the lateral sacral nodes, hypogastric, obturator and external iliac nodes.
Further spread is to the common iliac and para-aortic nodes. Lymph node
metastases in superficial tumours less than (TIIIA) are rare but if deep
muscle is involved the incidence of lymph node deposits is 20-30%. If
extravesical invasion is present 50-60% of patients have lymph node
metastases [17]. Haematogenous spread usually occurs late. The
predominant sites of metastases are the liver, bone and lungs.

MAGNETIC RESONANCE IMAGING

Technique

As with other imaging techniques a full bladder is essential to obtain
good quality images for the following reasons. First, the bladder tumour
is more likely to be identified when the bladder is full and second, a
full bladder displaces small bowel out of the pelvis thus diminishing
artefacts from bowel movement. In addition, errors due to
misinterpretation of small bowel loops lying adjacent to the bladder are
reduced. Most of the published data on MRI imaging of the bladder has
been carried out using superconductive low field systems (0.3 to 0.5
Tesla). In our Institute a high field Siemens Magnetom System (2 Tesla
operating at 1.5 Tesla) has been installed. Both T1-weighted and
T2-weighted sequences are required for examination of patients with
bladder cancer. The precise sequences used depend on the field strength
and type of scanner but, in general, sequences range as follows:-
T1-weighted (TR 300-800 ms, TE 15-35 ms), T2-weighted (TR 1500-2100 ms, TE
90-120 ms). New sequences are continually being developed for different
machines. For example, we are now using a new sequence for T1-weighted
images (TE 17 ms). One cm thick slices are obtained in the axial plane
with a 0-1 cm gap, we use a 5 mm gap. Following the initial T1 and
T2-weighted sequences in the axial plane additional scans are obtained in
the sagittal or coronal planes depending on the position of the primary

tumour. For example, tumours at the bladder base are elegantly displayed
on sagittal images.

The cylindrical body coil is routinely used but surface coils,
particularly the helmholtz type of coil, may be valuable for studying
pelvic tumours.

Normal appearances

On T1-weighted images the bladder appears as a low intensity structure
similar to that of the bladder wall. On T2-weighted images the urine has
a high intensity and with this sequence the bladder wall can therefore be
easily distinguished both from urine and from perivesical fat (Fig. 1 a &
b). The prostate and seminal vesicles, closely related to the base of the
bladder, are seen as low intensity structures on T1-weighted sequences but
the seminal vesicles have a higher intensity on T2-weighted sequences
(Fig. 1 a & b). The external iliac vessels and numerous other vessels
within the pelvis usually appear as low intensity structures because of
the 'flow void' phenomenon. Occasionally they are seen as bright, high
intensity, structures due to 'even echo rephasing' [18]. Normal lymph
nodes are not identified with MRI. Artefacts in pelvic scans are due to
movement and to chemical shift. Chemical shift artefacts occur at
water/fat interfaces, for example the interface between the bladder and
perivesical fat. Using low field systems chemical shift artefacts are
less of a problem than with high field systems. The artefact is seen as a
dark band along one side of the bladder and a bright band along the
opposite wall. With high field systems chemical shift artefact is also
seen along the small pelvic vessels around the prostate and bladder base.
These difficulties can significantly reduce information derived from MRI
images using high field systems.

Abnormal appearances in bladder cancer

Bladder tumours can be identified on MRI provided they are at least 1-2 cm
in diameter [19]. On T1-weighted sequences a bladder tumour appears as a
relatively low intensity mass compared with fat but of higher intensity
than urine (Fig. 2a). On T2-weighted sequences a bladder tumour has a
higher intensity than the normal bladder wall (Fig. 2b). It has been
suggested that deep muscle invasion can be distinguished from superficial
tumours by virtue of disruption of the low intensity line of the normal
bladder wall. Lee and his colleagues [20] demonstrated disruption of the
bladder wall in five out of eight patients with proven deep muscle tumour
spread (TIIIA). In nine patients with superficial tumours (no muscle
invasion), eight had an intact bladder wall in this series.

Spread of bladder cancer in to the perivesical fat (Stage TIIIB) is best
shown on T1-weighted images because there is high contrast between the low
intensity tumour and high intensity fat. Coronal and sagittal sections
are useful for demonstrating extravesical spread in patients with tumours
lying on the lateral and posterior bladder walls. Tumour spread into
adjacent organs such as the prostate and seminal vesicles may also be best
appreciated on coronal and sagittal images. Since the seminal vesicles
appear brighter than fat on T2-weighted sequences it is possible that
tumour invasion is shown best on T2-weighted images rather than on
T1-weighted sequences.

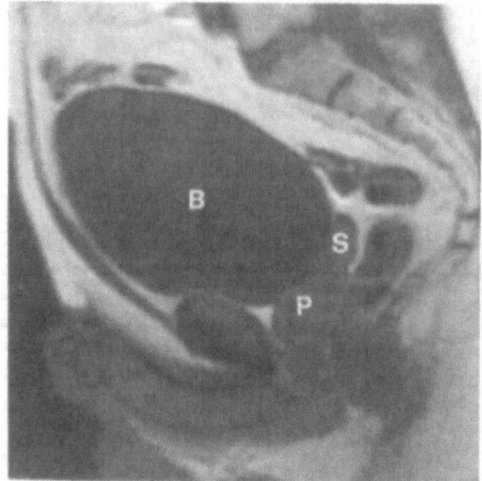

a

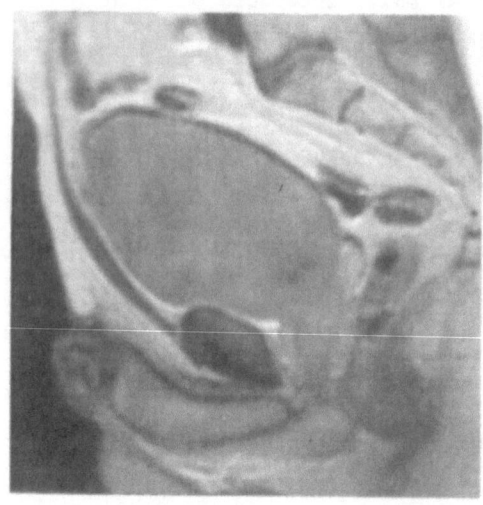

b

Fig. 1.   Sagittal sections through the pelvis.

    a.   T1-weighted sequence (TR 0.8, TE30). The bladder lumen (B) is
           seen as a low intensity structure as are the prostate (P) and
           seminal vesicles (S).

    b.   T2-weighted sequence (TR 2.1, TE 70). Urine in the bladder has
           a high intensity. Note seminal vesicles are also of high
           intensity.

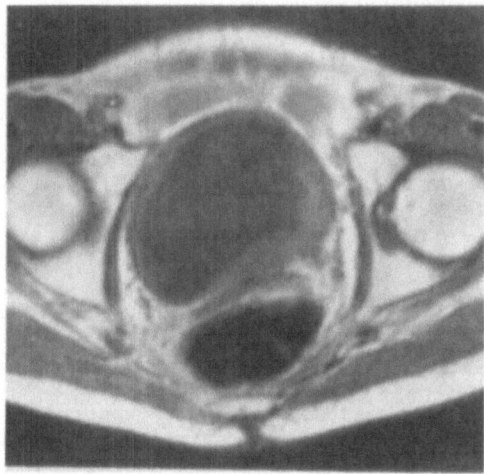

a

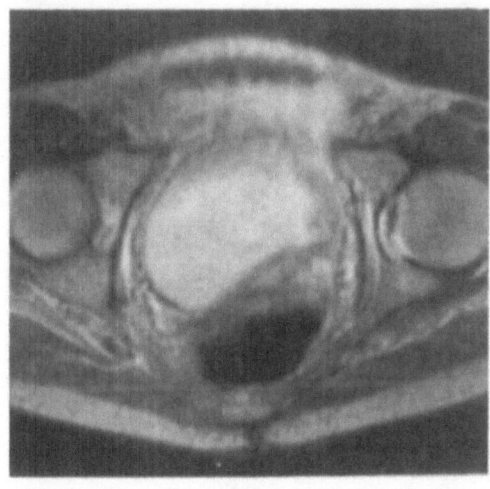

b

Fig. 2.   Tumour occupies the left lateral and posterior
           bladder walls.
      a.   On the T1-weighted sequence (TR 0.8, TE 30) it is seen as a
           higher intensity mass compared with urine.
      b.   On the T2-weighted sequence it has a lower intensity.

182

Enlarged lymph nodes have been demonstrated satisfactorily with MRI but
the same constraints regarding criteria for diagnosing lymph node
metastases apply to MRI as with CT. Thus enlargement is the only sign of
abnormality and lymphadenopathy due to reactive hyperplasia cannot be
distinguished from that due to malignant disease. Following endoscopy,
transurethral resection or radiotherapy MRI images are difficult to
interpret and similar limitations apply to MRI as to CT. Thus, mucosal
oedema, inflammation and blood clot cannot be distinguished from tumour on
the basis of signal intensity and thickening of the bladder wall due to
irradiation fibrosis cannot be reliably distinguished from persistent or
recurrent active tumour.

ACCURACY OF MRI

At present there are no large prospective series comparing MRI with
surgical staging in bladder cancer. However, small groups of patients
have been studied with both MRI and CT and preliminary results reported
[19,21,22,23]. Fisher and her colleagues [19] studied 14 patients in whom
comparison with CT was available in 11. MRI understaged two patients but
no patient was overstaged. In their comparison three out of 11 patients
were incorrectly staged using CT.

Bryan et al [22] correctly identified the presence or absence of
extravesical spread of tumour in 10 out of 13 patients with MRI, two being
understaged and one overstaged. With CT, staging was correct in nine of
the 13 patients. Three of these errors were due to understaging and one
due to overstaging. The patient who was overstaged with both techniques
had previously undergone a partial cystectomy. In this series three
patients had involved pelvic nodes. Lymphadenopathy was detected by both
MRI and CT in two out of the three patients. In this report Bryan et al
[22] concluded that MRI is a more accurate method of staging than CT, but
similar to CT has the inability to identify muscle invasion when the
tumour is confined to the bladder wall. This is in contra-distinction to
the views of Fisher and her colleagues [19] who suggest that Stage II
tumours should be distinguishable from Stage IIIA on the basis of
disruption of the low intensity bladder wall.

Amendola et al [21] have reported their experience of a comparison of MRI
with CT in 11 patients who underwent radical cystectomy including pelvic
lymph node dissections. They overstaged three patients with MRI and five
with CT, whereas understaging was only seen in one patient with each
modality. These authors agree with Bryan et al [22] that MRI is unable to
differentiate superficial T2 tumours from deep muscle invasion (TIIIA).
In this series two patients had lymph node metastases. Abnormal nodes
were identified by MRI in one of these patients but CT was not carried
out.

Recently, Rholl et al [23] have reported their experience in 23 patients.
MRI was correct in 22 out of 23 patients and CT in 16 out of 19 patients.
These authors found that MRI was an accurate method of determining bladder
integrity in the majority of patients. Thus, in six patients in whom the
bladder wall appeared disrupted on MRI, five had deep muscle invasion on
histology and of eight patients in whom the bladder wall appeared intact,
six had not evidence of muscle invasion and two had evidence of
superficial muscle invasion only on histology.

At the Royal Marsden Hospital we are also undertaking a prospective study comparing MRI and CT for staging bladder cancer. As yet the number of patients studied in whom histological verification is available is only ten and it is premature to discuss these results in details. Our study is being carried out using a Siemens High Field Strength Magnet of 1.5 and chemical shift artefacts cause considerable problems. The techniques appear equally accurate although on occasion extravesical spread is elegantly demonstrated with MRI.

All these authors conclude that MRI is more accurate than CT for staging bladder cancer. However, comparisons with CT have been carried out in small numbers of patients and large prospective series are required before any significant advantage of MR becomes apparent.

CONCLUSIONS

MRI is a promising new technique for evaluation of patients with bladder cancer. If the preliminary results discussed in this paper are substantiated in large series of patients then MRI may be particularly valuable for determining the integrity of the bladder wall and tumour invasion of the prostate and seminal vesicles. However, limitations of MRI are observed which are similar to those of CT. These include the inability to distinguish inflammation and oedema following cystoscopy from tumour and to distinguish irradiation fibrosis from residual disease within the bladder wall.

If the preliminary results regarding the accuracy of MRI are substantiated in large series of patients then the technique is likely to have an important place in staging bladder cancer.

REFERENCES

1.   Oliver R T D, Hendry W F, Bloom H J G. Overview and conclusions. In BLADDER CANCER, Butterworths, London. 1981, p.311
2.   Narayana A S, Loening S A, Slymen D J, Culp D A. Bladder cancer: factors affecting survival. J Urol 1983; 130: 56
3.   Bagshaw M A, Ray G R, Pistenma D A et al. External beam radiation therapy of primary carcinoma of the prostate. Cancer 1975; 36: 723
4.   Ray G R, Cassady J R, Bagshaw M A. External beam megavoltage radiation therapy in the treatment of post-radical prostatectomy residual or recurrent tumour: preliminary results. J Urol 1975; 114: 98
5.   Pilepich M V, Perez C A. Does radiotherapy alter the course of genitourinary cancer? In GENITOURINARY CANCER 1. Paulson D F (Ed). Martinus Nihoff, Boston. 1982, 215–238
6.   Silverberg E. Cancer Statistics 1983. CA 1983; 33: 9–25
7.   Byar D P, Mostofi F K. Carcinoma of the prostate: prognostic evaluation of certain pathologic features in 208 radical prostatectomies: examined by the step-section technique. Cancer 1972; 30: 5
8.   Jewett H J. The present status of radical prostatectomy for Stages A and B prostatic cancer. Urol Clin N Am 1975; 1: 105
9.   Richie J P, Skinner D G, Kaufmann J J. Carcinoma of the bladder: treatment by radical cystectomy. J Surg Res 1975; 18: 271

10. Ray G R, Pistenma D, Castellino R A et al. Operative staging of apparently localised adenocarcinoma of the prostate. Results in 50 unselected patients. Cancer 1976; 38: 73
11. Hodson N J, Husband J E, Macdonald J S. The role of computed tomography in the staging of bladder cancer. Clin Radiol 1979; 30: 389
12. Morgan C L, Calkins R F, Cavalcanti E J. Computed tomography in the evaluation, staging and therapy of carcinoma of the bladder and prostate. Radiology 1981; 140: 751
13. Vock P, Haertel M, Fuchs W A et al. Computed tomography in staging of carcinoma of the urinary bladder. Br J Urol 1982; 54: 158–163
14. Jewett H J, Strong G H. Infiltrating carcinoma of the bladder. J Urol 1946; 55: 365
15. Marshall V F. The relation of pre-operative estimate to the pathologic demonstration of the extent of vesical neoplasms. J Urol 1952; 68: 714
16. UICC (International Union Against Cancer). Harmer M H (ed). TNM Classification of Malignant Tumours. 3rd Ed. International Union Against Cancer, Geneva. 1978
17. van der Werf-Messing B, Schroeder F H, Bush H. Bladder. In TEXTBOOK OF CANCER. Halnan K E (ed). Chapman and Hall, London. 1982, p.457
18. Bradley W G, Waluch V. Blood flow: magnetic resonance imaging. Radiology 1985; 154: 443–450
19. Fisher M R, Hricak H, Tanagho E A. Urinary bladder MR imaging. II. Neoplasm. Radiology 1985; 157: 471–477
20. Lee J K T, Rholl K S, Heiken J P et al. Staging of bladder neoplasms by MRI. Presented at the Scientific Assembly and Annual Meeting of the Radiological Society of North America, Chicago 1985
21. Amendola M A, Glazer G M, Grossman H B, Aisen A M, Francis I R. Staging of bladder carcinoma: MR-CT-Surgical Correlation. AJR 1986; 146: 1179–1183
22. Bryan P J, Butler H E, LiPuma J P, Resnick M I, Kursh E D. CT and MR imaging in staging bladder neoplasms. J Comp Assist Tomogr 1987; 11: 96–101
23. Rholl K S, Lee J K T, Heiken J P, Ling D, Glazer H S. Primary bladder carcinoma: evaluation with MR imaging. Radiology 1987; 163: 117–121

PEDIATRIC MRI

PETER P.G.KRAMER.

INTRODUCTION
There are only a few review-articles in the literature on Magnetic
Resonance Imaging (MRI) in infants and children (14,12) and there is only
one book dealing with this subject (15), in spite of the fact that MRI is a
powerful image modality that is safe and painless and has a great potential
to become an important imaging modality in infants and children.In 1986 Cohen gives in his review (14) a description of the current status of MRI in
Pediatrics in that time, after referring to 115 articles in the literature
dealing in a greater or lesser extend with children. After 1985 many more
articles came into press and it seems that MRI establish itself as a
modality of choice for many clinical situations. There is no doubt that MRI
is the modality of choice in abnormalities in the central nervous system
and in musculoskeletal disorders. In other areas there still has to be done
more research for estimating the real place of MRI in the diagnostic tree.
In the next pages we will give you the state of the art of using MRI in
diseases in infants and children and give you our experiences and procedures in the University Hospital and the University Hospital for children and
youth in Utrecht, the Netherlands, where we have a Philips Gyroscan of 1.5
Tesla since August 1986.
Because MRI is a safe method without any known risk for children (even in
the cases of surgical clips, artificial heart valves, etc.) we can use MRI
from prenatal to adolescent age. There are articles dealing with the
anatomy and abnormalities in the intra uterine body. The examination of the
intracerebral myeliniation in preterm and term infants is subject to research with very detailed results. Also the existence and consequences of
hemorrhage and infarction/hypoxia in the neonatal brain is studied very
intensively.(40,47,48,49,50).
And so can we go on in age and find MRI used in many diseases and disorders.

Besides the advantages of MRI (safe, no radiation, non invasive, no discomfort, any body plane, superior soft tissue contrast resolution to CT,
spectroscopy posibilities) there are also some disadvantages like costs,
long scantime (30 - 60 min.), sensitive to motion, less sensitive for
calcification, slices bigger than 2 mm., problems with implanted magnetic
material. For these disadvantages it is necessary to prepare the patients
well and to choice the right indication for the examination.

PATIENT PREPARATION.
1. Explane the procedure carefully to the patient and the parents, if
possible by using photographs.
Like any X-ray department , a MRI room is also an anxious place for a child
(big machine, half-dark, noisy, etc.).

It is essential for the parents and for the child, if he/she can understand it, to tell them that there will be no pain, no injections, no catheters etc.

2. The child has to lay still for many minutes (30 - 60 min.). It depends of the age of the child which measures you can take to make the child feel comfortable or make it immobile. Parents stay close to the patient and are asked to read or tell stories.

3. A small infant has to be fed just prior to the examination.

4. If possible, in small infants but certain in bigger infants and children, the bladder should be emptied.

5. They all have to lay comfortable: supine, arms stretched beside the body, and warm. Newborns and small infants can be packed in a towel to prevent motion and to warmth them. ("let them feel back in utero"). Children from about 1 year to 4 to 5 years old give the most problems in immobilisation. Our experience with parents joining the child in the magnet is not hopeful. We do not use this method anymore. It is better to give sedation in individual cases. You can use the drug you are familiar with, for example:
-Chloral hydrate: 50 - 75 (100) mg/kg of body weight (orally) or,
-Sodium pentobarbital(Nembutal): 5 - 6 mg./kg. of body weight
 (intramuscullary or intravenously) 20 minutes prior to the
 examination (68).

Up to now our own experiences are the best with:
in-patients: a cocktail, intramuscullary, containing:
                - Pethidine Hydrochloride: 2 mg/kg B.W. (max. 40 mg.)
                - Chlorpromazine Hydrochloride: 0.5 mg/kg B.W.
                - Promethazine Hydrochloride: 0.5 mg/kg B.W.
out-patients: (sometimes also used for in-patients).
                - chloral hydrate: 60 - 75 mg/kg B.W. (max.
                  2500 mg.)
                - after 45 min., if necessary, a surplus
                  of 30 mg/kg B.W.

In about 10 percent of our exminations in the age group of 1 to 5 years, we have not optimal examinations, but in most cases we still can answer the questions of the clinicians. In very few cases it is really impossible to make any M.R. image of the child.

Up to now we do not use ventilators in the MRI examination-room because we do not have these equipment. And because the fact that our MRI equipment is placed in a new hospital, that will be opened in 1989, we can not examine children with a high risk. Also in literature, there are very few articles dealing with critical ill children.

MONITORING.
We only use visual monitoring of the child by the parents, nurses or the doctor who are with the child in the examination-room. Up to now we have not had any problem with that. But that depends on the selection of the patients who are coming for MRI. In literature we found some articles on the possibilities of monitoring equipment without ferrous metal. MR--compatible monitors for evaluation of body temperature, heartrate, bloodpressure, heart-ausculation and respiration (23,46,63) are available now, but still there is few experience, and we still do not have them.

COILS.
Use always the smallest coil as possible. Many parts of the body fit into the headcoil until approximately the age of 8 years. In some institution there are made special head and surface coils for children. We know from Bydder, G.M., London (personal communication) that he made the coils himself. We still have problems with finding the best coil for use in very small children and for superficial examination like the hand etc.

CONTRASTMEDIA.
We have not found articles inwhich contrastmedia are used in infants and small children. In the future it will be possible, also in small children, to use contrastmedia in examination for different organsystems like ferrite particles for bowel contrast (31), reticular endothelial system or liver etc.; Gadolineum-DTPA for intravenous administration etc. Hajek et al. (32) evaluated the potential contrast agents for MR arthrography inwhich Gadolineum-DTPA probably offers more advantages than others.

We shall now give you some remarks from the literature and our own results of the use of MRI in different organ systems. We only give a review from the literature of 1986 and the first half year of 1987. The literature up to 1985 is very well reviewed by Cohen (14).

CENTRAL NERVOUS SYSTEM.
As in adults, MRI is the modality of choice for evaluating the brain and the spinal medulla in infants and children. Because we can immediately make frontal, coronal, sagital and tranvers imaging of every part of the central nervous system. Because the pediatric brain matures during aging the relaxation characteristics change also. Nowell (55) described the difficulties in imaging these changing tissues. The best imaging she get was with a long SE sequences with a repetition time of 3000-3500 msec. and multiple echoes with the longest echo time of 120-160 msec.
Not only technical results are described, but also the anatomic differentiation. Nowadays radiologists are very interested in the development of the neonatal brain (40,47,48,49,50). The evaluation of periventricular leukomalacia with MRI is very well described by Wilson and Steiner (71). They found that MRI was able to depict the extent and progression of myelination, and it may be used to continue follow-up of these patients beyond the time of fontanel closure. Neoplasms and cysts in MR are already very well described in earlier years. MRI is an excellent noninvasive "screening" technique for children with suspected spinal cord disease and may be the only study needed in many patients with congenital spinal cord anomalies. It is also an excellent means to diagnose and follow patients with other forms of intra- and extraspinal pathology (57). Williams (70) described the possibility of the differentiation of intramedullary neoplasms and cysts. Also in the region of the sella MR proved to be more precise than CT (41). From the neurosurgical point of view MR proved to be superior or equivalent to other imaging technics (34). This was also true for follow-up studies after neurosurgical intervention (36).

MUSCULOSKELETAL SYSTEM.
Also in this system MR is the modality of choice because there is a superior soft-tissue visualisation (16). In the bones, cortex and bone marrow are very well devined. The soft-tissue examination is important in trauma, tumor and infection. It is very often superior to CT and nucleair medicine examination. About the validity of MR in Perthes disease is written very

much. Also when the plain radiograph is negative MR showes abnormalities that correlate to the appearance of vascular necroses. (35,45,52,53,69). Although investigated in adults, Beltran (8) was not able to distinguish fresh blood from saline in the knee joints. MR is highly sensitive for detecting fluid in the hip joint (51).

Dietrich et al. (19) described the MR imaging of the head and neck in the pediatric patients. They found that all entities were well delineated by MR imaging. Midline lesions were best imaged in the sagittal plane, lesions of paired structures and the face in the axial or coronal planes, and nasopharyngeal and oropharyngeal lesions in the axial or sagittal planes. Intracranial extension of head and neck neoplasms was best evaluated in the coronal plane. T2-weighted images provided better differentiation between normal and tumor tissue in patients with head and neck neoplasms. For bone marrow examination MRI is also a modality of choice. It is not possible to differentiate between various bone marrow disorders having a similar degree of cellularity (56). Bone marrow abnormalities are found in leukemia (54), neuroblastoma and sarcoma (10) etc.

There is also interest in MR imaging of spinal dysraphism (2,62). It is shown that MRI is a reliable technique for the initial evaluation in this abnormality.

Cartilage abnormalities as in juvenile chronic arthritis is another topic of MRI research. Also congenital dysplasia of the hip is, in difficult cases, a subject for MRI. For routinely examination we think that ultrasound will be a better and easier approach.

CARDIOVASCULAR SYSTEM.

In other chapters of this book cardiac MR will discuss in detail. An overview of MRI of the heart is given by Higgins (38), and in a paper about congenital heart disease which gated MR imaging by Didier (18). Coarctation of the aorta is also an abnormality which can be imaged by MR (4,42,64). But also in other congenital abnormalities of the great arteries MR is a exellent method of imaging (26). Evaluation of transplant candidates as, for example, the portal vein evaluation in pediatric liver transplant candidates is described by Day (17). We think that in the future MR of the great vessels and also minor vessels will be of great importancy, especial when contrastmedia can be used in children. Evaluation of vessels is also of great importancy in oncology. (see there).

ABDOMEN.

Gastrointestinal tract.

Bowel loops are not well identified by MRI. We think that for the abdomen CT is superior to MRI. Nevertheless all structures in the abdomen, except the bowel loops, can be identified well by MRI. All of that is well described in literature. The biggest problem in MRI of the abdomen is motion from respiration, cardiac pulsations, aorta pulsations and bowel peristalsis, of which respiration is the most important. Nowadays and in the future there will be developed fast imaging techniques that will overcome these difficulties. Respiratory gating has the disadvantage for increasing examination time. Steudel et al. (67) described a fast MR tomography of the liver inwhich fast field echo sequences are used. These authors gave also parameters for different measurements in liver diagnosis. Although not specific written on children Ferrucci (25) gave in the Leo J. Rigler Lecture "MRI Imaging of the liver" a superb review of the possibilities of MRI in liver diagnostics. In an article by Dietrich et al. (22) is described the possibility to demonstrate by MRI a wide spectrum of pelvic and perineal lesions, like congenital abnormalities, cystic lesions, fluid collections and neoplasma. In most of the described abnormalities MRI was superior to CT and ultrasound. Also MRI of the spleen, which has relatively long T1 and T2 relaxation times, makes it possible to differentiate between normal and abnormal like in sickle- cell anemia, were abnormally diminished signal intensity is seen (1). Also infarction and iron deposition can be seen easily. In 1986 and 1987 we did not found any new article about MRI of the pancreas. MRI is not routinily used for pancreas evaluation. In cystic fibrosis the pancreas is normal or small, while in pancreatitis the gland is enlarged which increased T1 and T2 relaxation times. What is also of interest is the MRI of the undescended testes. Gòmez Leòn (30) showed that CT is an accurate noninvasive method for detection of undescended testes, but Fritzsche (28) showed that MRI promised to become an important diagnostic tool in the detection of this abnormality. Also in other pathologic abnormalities of the scrotum MRI seems to become very important (3,60).

Genitourinary system.
   Kidney, ureter, bladder etc. can well be deliniate by MRI. The use of MRI in children with possible renal diseases is limited (20) and probably will ultrasonography and other X-ray modalities be the modality of choice.
   In renal transplants MRI can play a role in the evaluation of rejection. (5,33). Also in these problems MRI will be one of the tools inwhich ultrasonography probably is the modality of choice, besides scintigraphy. (39).
(Wilms' tumor see later).

CHEST
   Very few is written on the chest and mediastinum in children. Most of the articles reviewed by Cohen (14) are of adult patients. One of the first articles was of Brasch et al. (11). After that Laurin et al. (43)) gave also his initial experience and find that spatial resolution was slightly less with MRI than with CT. Medium and large vessels are well seen without contrastmedium injection. Tissue characterization with MRI is superior to CT and the normal thymus is well seen. On the other hand Siegel et al. (65) in his article on mediastinal lesions in children, compared MRI with CT. CT and MR provided comparable information regarding the presence and size of the mediastinal lesions, especially when a T1-weighted spin-echo pulse sequence was used. MR discriminated mediastinal masses and enlarged nodes from vascular structures and was more sentitive than CT in detecting intraspinal extension. They concluded that MRI may be more helpful than CT in evaluating posterior mediastinal tumors, since there is a likelihood of intraspinal extension. In other cases, however, CT continues to be the procedure of choice to supplement plain radiography in children with suspected mediastinal neoplasms. MR Imaging of the chest is capable of demonstrating airway obstruction in infants and delineating any relationship to major mediastinal blood vessels (26). The chest radiograph is still the major modality for studying the lungs, but MRI can be helpful in differentiating pathology.

RETICULOENDOTHELIAL AND ENDOCRINE DISORDERS.
   As already described by Cohen in 1986 (14) enlarged lymph nodes are easy to identify with MR. He gives also a good overview in the possibilities of enlarged lyphoma in different diseases, and that MRI could not distinguish between the different histological types of lymphoma (13).
   The thymus is easily visible and differed from subcutaneous fat in hydrogen density. The T1 relaxation times of the thymus (mean = 703 msec.)

were much longer than those of fat in patients under 30 years of age. MR may be better than CT is distinguishing between thymus replaced by fat and mediastinal fat (29).

The marked prolongation of relaxation times associated with thyroid disease causes excellent contrast of lesions with normal thyroid and surrounding structures, as found by Higgins et al. (37), who studied the thyroid gland in adult patients. I did not found any articel on MR imaging the thyroid in children.

ONCOLOGY

Belt described in 1986 (7) the promise of MRI as the primary imaging method for Wilms' Tumor identification. Magnetic resonance accurately identified the primary tumor and its renal origin in all cases, and tumor margins and local extensions were accurately demonstrated. Nevertheless some surgical proven instances of capsular invasion were missed. Metastatic spread into the liver and inferior vena cava was well documented or excluded in all cases. All Wilms' Tumors had signal intensities consistent with prolonged T1 and T2 relaxation times. Signal intensity was highly variable, mainly because of necrosis and hemorrhage within the tumor. Magnetic resonance has the potential for providing the same information as computed tomography, sonography, liver spleen radionuclide scanning, and excretory urography.

Dietrich (21) described that MR appears to be a reliable technique for the diagnosis, staging, and follow-up of children with neuroblastoma. It accurately detected the lesions and their extent in all patients. It correctly evaluated the possibility of resectability and showed metastases, response to treatment and development of complications.

MR may also be useful for distinguishing extrahepatic cavernous hemangiomas from other soft-tissue tumors, particularly sarcomas (44).

ARTIFACTS.

As in adults one must care about artifacts mostly caused by motion. But also other artifacts did rises from the process of creating a MR image. Last years there are written some perfect reviews on these artifacts, variants, and other factors degrating image quality, also in pediatric magnetic resonance imaging (6,58,59,61,66).

CONCLUSION.

We hope that we make clear that MR imaging has a great potential to become an important image modality in infants and children. In some areas (see central nervous system, musculoskeletal disorders etc.) MRI is the modality of choice. In other area we still have to do more research to get more information about the sensitivity and specificity of MRI. Also the inpact on therapy has to be investigated very sharply. If we have this information we can estimate the real place of MRI in the diagnosis of diseases and abnormalities in children.

ACKNOWLEDGMENTS.

The author wish to thank Th.D. Witkamp, M.D., radiologist and J.H.W. van 't Hout, M.D. for assistance, and Grace van Schaik for manuscript preparation.

191

References.

For a review of the literature up to 1985 see Cohen 1986 (14).

1. Adler DD, Glazer GM, Aisen AM: MRI of the spleen: Normal Appearance and Findings in Sickle-Cell Anemia. AJR 1986; 147:843-845.
2. Altman NR, Altman DH: MR Imaging of Spinal Dysraphism. AJNR 1987; 8:533-538.
3. Baker LL, Hajek PC, Burkhard TK, Dicapua L, Landa HM, Leopold GR, Hesselink JR, Mattrey RF: MR Imaging of the Scrotum Pathologic Conditions. Radiology 1987; 163:93-98.
4. Bank ER, Aisen AM, Rocchinni AP, Hernandez RJ: Coarctation of the Aorta in Children Undergoing Angioplasty: Pretreatment and Posttreatment MR Imaging. radiology 1987; 162:235-240.
5. Baumgartner BR, Nelson RC, Ball, TI, Wyly JB, Bourke E, Delaney V, Bernardino ME: MR Imaging of Renal Transplants. AJR 1986; 147:949-953.
6. Bellon EM, Haacke EM, Coleman PE, Sacco DC, Steiger DA, Gangarosa RE: MR Arfifacts: A Review. AJR 1986; 147:1271-1281.
7. Belt TG, Cohen MD, Smith JA, Cory DA, McKenna S, Weetman R: MRI of Wilms' Tumor: Promise as the Primary Imaging Method. AJR 1986; 146:955-961.
8. Beltran J, Noto AM, Herman LJ, Mosure JC, Burk JM, Christoforidis AJ: Joint Effusions: MR Imaging. Radiology 1986; 158:133-137.
9. Benz-Bohm G, Widemann B, Herrmann F, Weidtman V: Ist die Hüftsonographie als Screeningsuntersuchung sinnvoll? Fortschr. Röntgenstr. 1987; 146,2:188-191.
10. Boyko OB, Cory DA, Cohen MD, Provisor A, Mirkin D, DeRosa GP: MR Imaging of Osteogenic and Ewing's Sarcoma. AJR 1987; 148:317-322.
11. Brasch RC, Gooding CA, Lallemand DP, Wesbey GE: Magnetic Resonance Imaging of the Thorax in Childhood. Radiology 1984; 150:463-467.
12. Brasch RC: Magnetic Resonance Imaging for Pediatric Diagnosis. Magnetic Resonance Annual 1987:179-201.
13. Cohen MD, Klatte EC, Smith JA, Martin-Simmerman P, Carr B, Baehner R, Weetman R, Provisor A, Coates T, Berkow R, Weiman SJ, McKenna S, McGuire W: Magnetic resonance imaging of lymphomas in children. Pediatr.Radiol. 1985; 15:179-183.
14. Cohen MD: Clinical Utility of Magnetic Resonance Imaging in Pediatrics. AJDS 1986; 140:947-956.
15. Cohen MD: Pediatric Magnetic Resonance Imaging. W.B. Saunders Company, Philadelphia, 1986.
16. Cohen MD, DeRosa GP, Kleiman M, Passo M, Cory DA, Smith JA, McKinney L: Magnetic Resonance Evaluation of Disease of the Soft Tissues in Children. Pediatrics 1987; 79,5:696-701.
17. Day DL, Letourneau JG, Allan BT, Ascher NL, Lund G: MR Evaluation of the Portal Vein in Pediatric Liver Transplant Candidates. AJR 1986; 147:1027-1030.
18. Didier D, Higgins CB, Fischer MR, Osaki L, Silverman NH, Cheitlin MD: Congenital Heart Disease: Gated MR Imaging in 72 Patients. Radiology 1986; 158:227-235.
19. Dietrich RB, Lufkin RB, Kangarloo H, Hanafee WN, Wilson GH: Head and Neck MR Imaging in the Pediatric Patient. Radiology 1986; 159:769-776.
20. Dietrich RB, Kangarloo H: Kidneys in Infants and Children: Evaluation with MR. Radiology 1986; 159:215-221.

21. Dietrich RB, Kangarloo H, Lenarsky C, Feig SA: Neuroblastoma: The Role of MR Imaging. AJR 1987; 148:937-942.
22. Dietrich RB, Kangarloo H: Pelvic Abnormalities in Children: Assessment with MR Imaging. Radiology 1987; 163:367-372.
23. Dunn V, Coffman CE, McGowan JE, Ehrhardt JC: Mechanical Ventilation During Magnetic Resonance Imaging. Magnetic Resonance Imaging 1985; 3,2:169-172.
24. Ehman RL, McNamara MT, Brasch RC, Felmlee JP, Gray JE, Higgins CB: Influence of Physiologic Motion on the Appearance of Tissue in MR Images. Radiology 1986; 159:77-782.
25. Ferrucci JT: MR Imaging of the Liver. AJR 1986; 147:1103-1116.
26. Fletcher BD, Dearborn DG, Mulopulos GP: MR Imaging in Infants with Airway Obstruction: Prelimary Observations. Radiology 1986; 160:245-249.
27. Fletcher BD, Jacobstein MD: MRI of Congenital Abnormalities of the Great Arteries. AJR 1986; 146:941-948.
28. Fritzsche PJ, Hricak H, Kogan BA, Winkler ML, Tanagno EA: Undescended Testis: Value of MR Imaging. Radiology 1987; 164:169-173.
29. Geer G de, Webb WR, Gamsu G: Normal Thymus: Assesment with MR and CT. Radiology 1986; 158:313-317.
30. Gòmez Leòn MN, Ferreiròs J, Casanova R, Rodriguez R, Pedrosa CS: The Value of Computed Tomography in the Localization of Undescended Testes. Europ.J.Radiol. 1986; 6:283-287.
31. Hahn PF, Stark DD, Saini S, Lewis JM, Wittenberg J, Ferrucci JT: Ferrite Particles for Bowel Contrast in MR Imaging: Design Issues and Feasibility Studies. Radiology 1987; 164:37-41.
32. Hajek PC, Sartoris DJ, Neumann CH, Resnick D: Potential Contrast Agents for MR Arthrography: In Vivro Evaluation and Practical Observations. AJR 1987; 149:97-104.
33. Halasz NA: Differential Diagnosis of Renal Transplant Rejection: Is MR Imaging the Answer? AJR 1986; 147:954-955.
34. Hanigan WC, Wright SM, Wright RM: Clinical Utility of Magnetic Resonance Imaging in Pediatric Neurosurgical Patients. J.Pediatr. 1986; 108:522-529.
35. Heuck A, Reiser M, Rupp N, Lehner K, Erlemann R: Die Darstellung der Femurkopfnekrose in der MR-Tomographie. Fortschr.Röntgenstr. 1987; 146,2:191-195.
36. Higer HP, Gutjahr P, Schmidberger P, Dittrich M, Pfannenstiel P: NMR Follow-Up Studies of CNS-Tumors in Infancy and Childhood. Europ.J.Radiol. 1987; 7:49-53.
37. Higgins CB, McNamara MT, Fisher MR, Clark OH: MR Imaging of the Thyroid. AJR 1986; 147:1255-1261.
38. Higgins CB: Overview of MR of the Heart-1986. AJR 1986; 146:907-918.
39. Hricak H, Terrier F, Marotti M, Engelstad BL, Filly RA, Vincenti F, Duca RM, Bretan PN, Higgins CB, Feduska N: Posttransplant Renal Rejection: Comparison of Quantitative Scintigraphy, US, and MR Imaging. Radiology 1987; 162:685-688.
40. Johnson MA, Pennock JM, Bydder GM, Dubowitz LMS, Thomas DJ, Young IR: Serial MR Imaging in Neonatal Cerebral Injury. AJNR 1987; 8:83-92.
41. Kalifa G, Demange Ph, Sellier N, LaLande G, Chaussain JL, Bennet J: Magnetic Resonance Imaging (MRI) of the Sellar and Juxtasellar Area in Children. Ann.Radiol. 1986; 29,8:669-673.

42. Kersting-Sommerhoff BA, Sechtem UP, Fisher MR, Higgins CB: MR Imaging of Congenital Anomalies of the Aortic Arch. AJR 1987; 149:9-13.
43. Laurin S, Williams JL, Fitzsimmons JR: Magnetic Resonance Imaging of the Pediatric Thorax: Initial Experience. Europ.J.Radiol. 1986; 6:36-41.
44. Levine E, Wetzel LH, Neff JR: MR Imaging and CT of Extrahepatic Cavernous Hemangiomas. AJR 1986; 147:1299-1304.
45. Markisz JA, Knowles RJR, Altchek DW, Schneider R, Whalen JP, Cahill PT: Segmental Patterns of Avascular Necrosis of the Femoral Heads: Early Detection with MR Imaing. Radiology 1987; 162:717-720.
46. McArdle CB, Nicholas DA, Richardson CJ, Amparo EG: Monitoring of the Neonate Undergoing MR Imaging: Technical Considerations. Radiology 1986; 159:223-226.
47. McArdle CB, Richardson CJ, Hayden CK, Nicholas DA, Crofford MJ, Amparo EG: Abnormalities of the Neonatal Brain: MR Imaging. Part I.Intracranial Hemorrhage. Radiology 1987; 163:387-394.
48. McArdle CB, Richardson CJ, Hayden CK, Nicholas DA, Amparo EG: Abnormalities of the Neonatal Brain: MR Imaging. Part II.Hypoxic-Ischemic Brain Injury. Radiology 1987; 163:395-403.
49. McArdle CB, Richardson CJ, Nicholas DA, Mirfakhraee M, Hayden CK, Amparo EG: Development Features of the Neonatal Brain: MR Imaging. Part I.Gray-White Matter Differentiation and Myelination. Radiology 1987; 162:223-229.
50. McArdle CB, Richardson CJ, Nicholas DA, Mirfakhraee M, Hayden CK, Amparo EG: Development Features of the Neonatal Brain: MR Imaging. Part II.Ventricular Size and Extracerebral Space. Radiology 1987;
51. Mitchell DG, Rao V, Dalinka M, Spritzer CE, Gefter WB, Axel L, Steinberg M, Kressel HY: MRI of Joint Fluid in the Normal and Ischemic Hip. AJR 1986; 146:1215-1218.
52. Mitchell DG, Joseph PM, Fallon M, Hickey W, Kressel HY, Rao VM, Steinberg ME, Dalinka MK: Chemical-Shift MR Imaging of the Femoral Head: An In Vitro Study of Normal Hips and Hips with Avascular Necrosis. AJR 1987; 148:1159-1164.
53. Mitchell DG, Rao VM, Dalinka MK, Spritzer CE, Alavi A, Steinberg ME, Fallon M, kressel HY: Femoral Head Avascular Necrosis: Correlation of MR Imaging, Radiographic Staging, Radionuclide Imaging, and Clinical Findings. Radiology 1987; 162:709-715.
54. Moore SG, Gooding CA, Brasch RC, Ehman Rl, Ringertz HG, Ablin AR, Matthay KK, Zoger S: Bone Marrow in Children with Acute Lymphocytic Leukemia MR Relaxation Times. Radiology 1986; 160:237-240.
55. Nowell MA, Hackney DB, Zimmerman RA, Bilaniuk LT, Grossman RI, Goldberg HI: Immature Brain: Spin-Echo Pulse Sequence Parameters for High-Contrast MR Imaging. Radiology 1987; 162:272-273.
56. Nyman R, Rehn S, Glimelius B, Hagberg H, Hemmingsson A, Jung B, Simonsson B, Sundström C: Magnetic Resonance Imaging in Diffuse Malignant Bone Marrow Diseases. Acta Radiologica 1987; 28:199-205.
57. Packer RJ, Zimmerman RA, Sutton LN, Bilaniuk LT, Bruce DA, Schut L: Magnetic Resonance Imaging of Spinal Cord Disease of Childhood. Pediatrics 1986; 78,2:251-256.
58. Patton JA, Kulkarni MV, Craig JK, Wolfe OH, Price RR, Partain CL, James AE: Techniques, pitfalls and artifacts in magnetic resonance imaging. Radiographics 1987; 7,3:505-519.
59. Porter BA, Hastrup W, Richardson Ml, Wesbey GE, Olson DO, Cromwell LD, Moss AA: Classification and investigation of artifacts in magnetic resonance imaging. Radiographics 1987; 7,2:271-287.

60. Rholl KS, Lee JKT, Ling D, Heiken JP, Glazer HS: MR Imaging of the Scrotum with a High-Resolution Surface Coil. Radiology 1987; 163:99-103.
61. Ringertz HG, Brasch RC, Gooding CA: Artifacts, variants, and factors degrading image quality in pediatric magnetic resonance imaging. Pediatr.Radiol. 1985; 15:173-178.
62. Roos RAC, Vielvoye GJ, Voormolen JHC, Peters ACB: Magnetic Resonance Imaging in Occult Spinal Dysraphism. Pediatr.Radiol. 1986; 16:412-416.
63. Roth JL, Nugent M, Gray JE, Julsrud PR, Berquist TH, Sill JC, Kispert DB: Patient Monitoring during Magnetic Resonance Imaging. Anesthesiology 1985; 62:80-83.
64. Schulthess GK, Higashino SM, Higgins SS, Didier D, Fisher MR, Higgins CB: Cardiovascular-Interventional Radiology. Coarctation of the Aorta: MR Imaging. Radiology 1986; 158,2:469-474.
65. Siegel MJ, Nadel SN, Glazer HS, Sagel SS: Mediastinal Lesions in Children: Comparison of CT and MR. Radiology 1986; 160:241-244.
66. Stark DD, Hendrick RE, Hahn PF, Ferrucci JT: Motion Artifact Reduction with Fast Spin-Echo Imaging. Radiology 1987; 164:183-191.
67. Steudel A, Träber F, Krahe T, Gieseke J, Lackner K, Thurn P: Schnelle MR-Tomographie der Leber. Fortschr.Röntgenstr. 1987; 147,1:51-57.
68. Strain JD, Harvey LA, Foley LC, Campbell JB: Intravenously Administered Pentobarbital Sodium for Sedation in Pediatric CT. Radiology 1986; 161:105-108.
69. Thickman D, Axel L, Kressel HY, Steinberg M, Chen H, Velchick M, Fallon M, Dalinka M: Magnetic Resonance Imaging of Avascular Necrosis of the Femoral Head. Skeletal Radiol. 1986; 15:133-140.
70. Williams AL, Haughton VM, Pojunas KW, Daniels DL, Kilgore DP: Differentiation of Intramedullary Neoplasms and Cysts by MR. AJR 1987; 149:159-164.
71. Wilson DA, Steiner RE: Periventricular Leukomalacia: Evaluation with MR Imaging. Radiology 1986; 160:507-511.

SECTION V MUSCULOSKELETAL IMAGING

MRI OF THE MUSCULOSKELETAL SYSTEM: NORMAL ANATOMY

G.J. KIEFT, J.L. BLOEM

MRI is a rapidly evolving diagnostic tool in the evaluation of musculoskeletal disease. Its advantage include absence of ionizing radiation, excellent tissue contrast, its lack of streak artifacts from cortical bone and the multiplanar imaging capability. This allows visualization of anatomic structures in more convenient planes than other methods such as computed tomography (CT).

CT like MRI provides delineation of bone, fat and soft tissue but the ability of CT in this last category is limited because the difference in X-ray attenuation values between normal and abnormal tissues is often minimal.

The potential of MRI as a non-invasive imaging modality of the musculoskeletal system seems good especially because anatomic detail of the spine and the appendicular skeleton can be visualized without motion artefacts. Recent refinements in imaging techniques such as surface coils (Fig. 1) with improved signal to noise ratio and examination of thinner slices with better spatial resolution will further establish MRI as a powerful diagnostic tool.

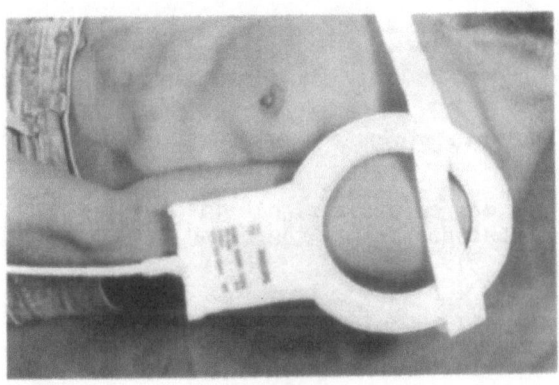

Fig. 1. Surface coil for the shoulder

Optimal pulse sequences

This discussion will be confined to the spin-echo imaging of the musculoskeletal system. Magnetic Resonance signal intensity is dependent on three tissue parameters, T1, T2 and hydrogen density and two instrument parameters: the repetition time (TR) and the echo time (TE). Each tissue has its own characteristic tissue parameters, the instrument parameters can be widely varied. These five parameters interact in a complex manner to produce a certain signal intensity for each tissue. Therefore pulse sequence optimization seems a difficult problem. However in practice we use a simple strategy, the relative intensities of most normal tissues are rather constant throughout most practical TR and TE combinations

198

(table I).
Pathologic tissue like edematous or inflammatory tissue, neoplastic tissue or joint effusion have significantly different intensity behaviour with changes in TR and TE. These tissues tend to have elevated values of T1 and T2 and therefore appear as low intensity areas on T1 weighted and as high intensity areas on T2 weighted images.

By using a combination of both T1 and T2 weighted images we will have adequate contrast between normal and abnormal tissue no matter what background tissue is involved.

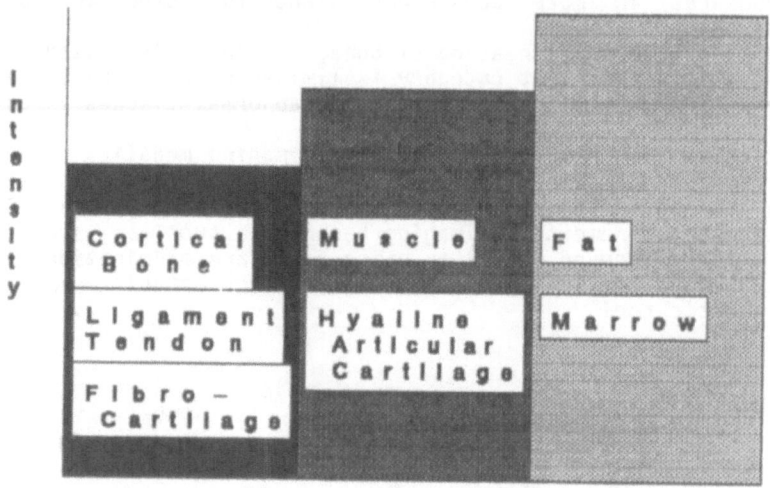

Table I. Relative intensities of most normal-musculoskeletal tissues.

Bone marrow
Adult yellow bone marrow has a signal intensity that is comparable to subcutaneous fat, because fat is composing the majority of the marrow volume in adults (Fig. 2).

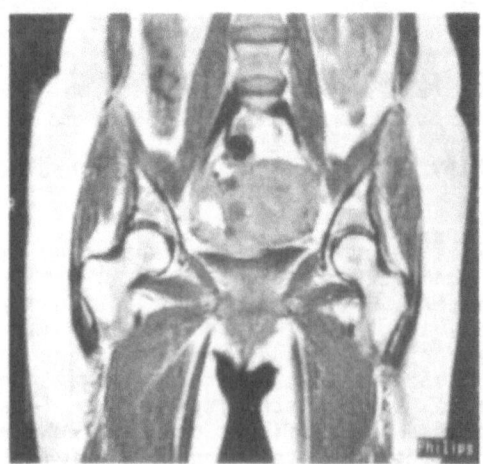

Fig. 2. Coronal T1 weighted image (TR 550, TE 30) of the proximal femora and pelvis of an adult.

Red hematopoietic bone marrow has an increased cellularity and therefore contains more water (longer T1) than yellow (fatty) marrow and will appear darker on T1 weighted images. Young children have a much more extensive distribution of red bone marrow than adults, therefore T1 weighted images in children will show a lower marrow signal than in adults except the femoral capital epifyses and greater trochanters, areas of normal yellow marrow (Fig. 3).

With increasing age red marrow recedes from the appendicular skeleton, during the middle of the third decade the adult red marrow distribution has been reached, with red marrow mainly found in the axial skeleton.

Trabecular patterns and normal epifysial lines can be seen as low signal intensity areas and should not be confused with areas of necrosis or fractures.

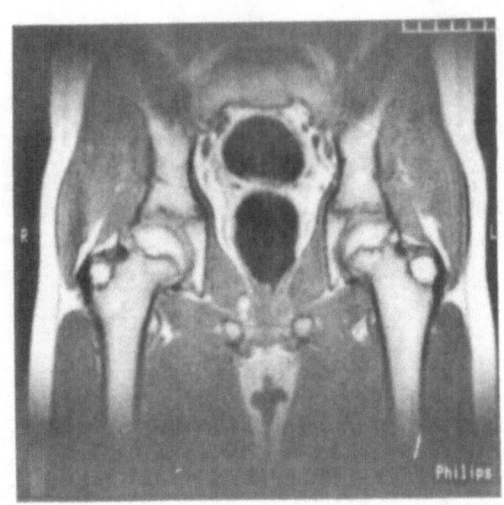

Fig. 3. Coronal T1 weighted image (TR 550, TE 30) of the proximal femora and pelvis of a child.

Normal anatomy of shoulder and knee, optimal image plane selection.

In recent literature several authors have described the normal MR appearances of some of the major joints including the hip, the knee and the shoulder. Imaging characteristics of the various articular tissues are similar among different joints (table I).

Figures 4 and 5 demonstrate these characteristics.

Important anatomic structures in shoulder and knee as the rotator cuff and cruciate ligaments are obliquely oriented. Oblique images for which the angulation is chosen on the transverse image allow optimal visualization of these structures. In the normal knee the medial and lateral collateral ligaments are silhouetted by fat and are best seen in the coronal plane. These ligaments will appear as low intensity linear structures against the high intensity background of fat (Fig. 4).

The posterior cruciate ligament is best identified in the sagittal plane, the 20 sagittal ligament is best identified in the sagittal plane,

the 20 sagittal image is best suited for visualization of the anterior
cruciate ligament (clock wise rotation for the left and counter clock wise
rotation for the right anterior cruciate ligament). Both ligaments can
well be visualized as homogeneous low signal intensity bands.

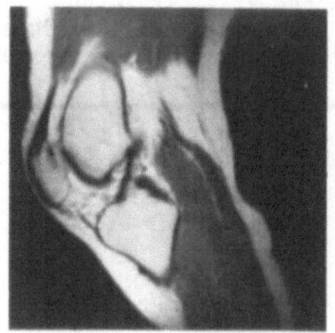 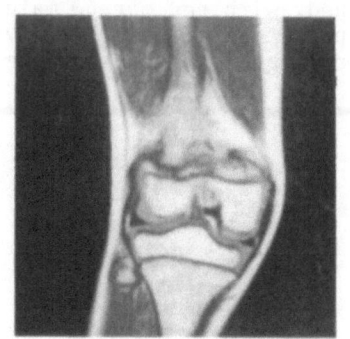

Fig. 4.
T1 weighted (TR 550, TE 30)
sagittal image of the knee, the anterior cruciate ligament is well visualized (arrow).

Fig. 5.
T1 weighted (TR 550, TE 30)
coronal image of the knee, both menisci can be seen as low intensity
triangular structures (arrows), there
is also a joint effusion.

The menisci can be seen on both coronal and sagital planes as low intensity triangular structures due to their fibrocartilage substance and
can be distinguished from the high intensity hyaline cartilage. When a
joint effusion is present the visualization is even better due to the
higher signal from the effusion on both T1 and T2 weighted images (Fig.
V).
In the shoulder joint stability is highly dependent on the soft tissues
like rotator cuff muscles and tendons and the glenoid labrum. The rotator
cuff muscles and tendons and their relationship to the coracoacromial arc
are best seen on oblique planes, parallel and longitudinally perpendicular
to the glenoid cavity.
The axial plane as well as the oblique plane longitudinally perpendicular to the glenoid is best suited for demonstration of the glenoid labrum
(Fig. VI).
In recent literature investigations on the use of MRI in other joints as
wrist, ankle and temporomandibular joint have been published. Much additional work will have to be performed before MRI becomes a standard diag-

nostic tool in these joints.

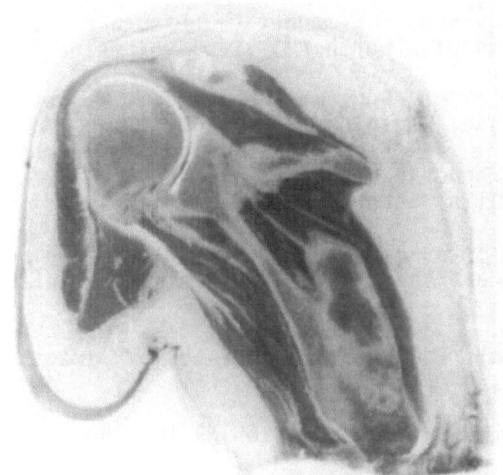 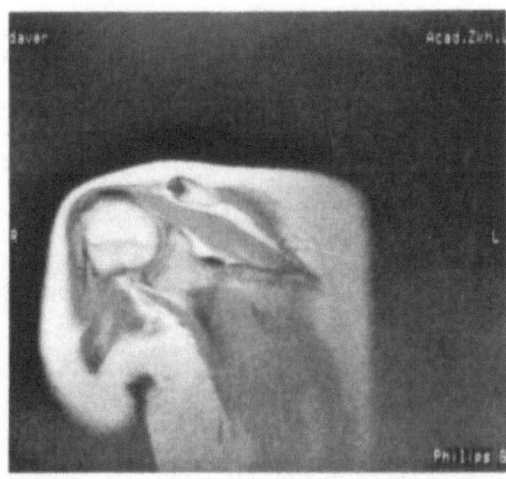

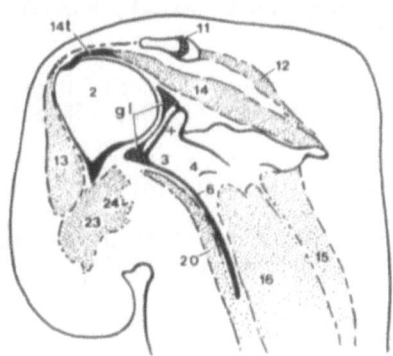

Fig. VI.
Section through the humeral head and scapula. The hyaline articular cartilage of both the glenoid cavity (+) and humeral head has a high signal
intensity, in contrast with the fibrous cartilage of the glenoid labrum
(gl). Notice the supraspinatus muscle (14), which is cut in its entire
length from origin to insertion (14t). (From G.J. Kieft, et al, Radiology
1986; 159: 741-745, reproduced with permission).

CONCLUSION
MRI is becoming increasingly important in the evaluation of articula-
tions and the skeleton, soft tissue anatomy can already be studied in
great detail, with further improvements in resolution, image acquisition
time, as well as experience in image interpretation MRI will probably become the most important non-invasive diagnostic tool in the evaluation of
the musculoskeletal system.

REFERENCES

1. Richardson ML. Optimizing pulse sequences for magnetic resonance imaging of the musculoskeletal system. Rad Clin North Am. 1986; vol 24:no 2.

2. Dooms GC, Fischer MR, Hricak H et al. Bone marrow imaging: Magnetic resonance studies related to age and sex. Radiology 1985; 155:429-432.

3. Jergesen HE, Heller M, Genant HK. Magnetic resonance imaging in osteo-necrosis of the femoral head. Orthop Clin North Am 1985; 16:664-694.

4. Littrup PJ, Aisen AM, Braunstein EM et al. Magnetic resonance imaging of femoral head development in radiographically normal patients. Skeletal Radiol 1984; 14:159-163.

5. Beltran J, Noto A, Mosure JC et al. The knee: Surface-coil MR imaging at 1.5 T. Radiology 1986; 159:747-751.

6. Gallimore GW, Harms SE. Knee injuries: High-resolution MR Imaging. Radiology 1986; 160:457-461.

7. Kieft GJ, Bloem JL, Obermann WR et al. Normal shoulder: MR Imaging. Radiology 1986; 159:741-745.

8. Middleton WD, Kneeland JB, Carrera JB et al. High resolution MR Imaging of the normal rotator cuff. Am J Radiol 1987; 148:559-564.

9. Kieft GJ, Sartoris DW, Bloem JL et al. Magnetic Resonance Imaging of gleno-humeral joint disease. Skeletal Radiol 1987; 16:285-290.

10. Li KC, Henkelman RM, Poon PY, Rubinstein J. MR Imaging of the normal knee. J Comput Assist Tomogr 1984; 6:1147-1154.

11. Sims RE, Genant HK. Magnetic Resonance Imaging of joint disease. Rad Clin North Am 1986 June; vol 24:no 2.

12. Roberts D, Schenck J, Joseph P et al. Temporo mandibular joint: magnetic resonance imaging. Radiology 1985; 115:829-830.

MRI OF MUSCULOSKELETAL DISEASE

J.L. BLOEM, A.H.M. TAMINIAU, R.M. BLOEM

INTRODUCTION

The role of MRI in diagnosis of musculoskeletal disease was at first considered to be very limited. The absence of signal from cortical bone was interpreted as a major disadvantage. In the past few years however interest and experience in MRI of musculoskeletal disease have expanded rapidly. Already MRI has an important place in diagnosis of musculoskeletal disease (1).

This chapter presents an overview of MRI applications in the musculoskeletal system excluding joint disease. The illustrations are with the exception of Figure 2 made with a 0.5 T Philips Gyroscan. So called T1 weighted images were made with SE technique TR 550, TE 30. T2 weighted images were made with SE technique TR 1500-2500, TE 50-100. Number of excitations per data time was four to six for T1 weighted images and two for T2 weighted images.

BONE MARROW DISEASE

Bone marrow can be directly visualized with good spatial resolution and with high contrast between normal and pathological marrow. Thus malignant infiltration of bone marrow can be detected before destruction of bone trabeculae occur. Bone marrow disorders including leukaemia, lymphoma, plasmocytoma, Paget's disease, osteomyelitis, osteopetrosis, Gaucher's disease, myelofibrosis and metastases can all be diagnosed with high sensitivity, because of the low signal intensity of these disorders on T1 weighted images (1,9,10,14) (Fig.1-5). High contrast between low signal intensity of tumor and high signal intensity of normal bone marrow facilitates detection (Fig.1).

The specificity of MRI is low. Most disorders have an identical low signal intensity. But as experience accumulates some specific MR signs emerge. As a rule T1 and T2 relaxation times as well as spin density are increased in pathological tissue. This pattern results in high signal intensity of pathological tissue on T2 weighted images and a low signal intensity on T1 weighted images (Fig.1-5). Exceptions to this common pattern may sometimes suggest a specific diagnosis. Osteopetrosis for instance is - because of a very low spin density - characterized by absence of signal on all pulse sequences. Uncomplicated Gaucher's disease has a relatively low signal intensity on T2 weighted images because of the paramagnetic effect of Gaucher cells. The low signal intensity on T2 weighted images may also represent secondary osteonecrosis. A high signal intensity on T2 weighted images is seen in secondary osteomyelitis or when an inflammatory reaction or venous congestion is present (Fig.4) (9). Osteoporosis does not change the signal intensity of marrow, because bone marrow is not replaced by other tissue. Therefore osteoporosis cannot be detected by MRI. By virtue of this insensitivity to osteoporosis, MRI can differentiate osteoporosis from marrow infiltrated by tumor. Osteoporotic fractures may thus be differentiated from tumor related fractures.

Transient ischaemic osteoporosis can be detected by MRI because it has the same MRI characteristics as osteomyelitis: a decreased signal intensity on T1 weighted images and an increased signal intensity on T2 weighted images. This is caused by the accompanying sterile inflammatory reaction in transient ischemic osteoporosis (Fig.5)

OSTEONECROSIS AND PERTHES DISEASE

Osteonecrosis is usually represented by a low signal intensity area on T1 and T2 weighted images (Fig.6) (8). The signal intensity may be increased on T1 or T2 weighted images due to inflammatory reaction and secondary hemorrhage. An increased signal intensity on T1 weighted images is also found when fatty marrow conversion precedes or accompanies osteonecrosis (11,12). Concomitant joint effusion is often seen on T2 weighted images. The subarticular localization of clinically important osteonecrosis increases specificity.

The sensitivity and specificity of MRI are reported to be higher than planar Tc-99m diphosphonate scintigraphy (12). Sometimes bilateral disease is detected by MRI in a patient with unilateral symptoms. So far all these patients progressed to bilateral clinical disease within three months. It is possible that not all patients with positive MRI signs develop symptomatic osteonecrosis because the low signal intensity seen on MRI reflects changes in bone marrow. Further research is needed to determine what percentage of clinically silent patients with MRI abnormalities progress to necrosis of bone itself. MRI may because of its high sensitivity in the early phase, play a role in the diagnosis of osteonecrosis initiated by a fracture. This may be important in planning conservative or surgical treatment.

MRI as a non-invasive, non-ionizing imaging modality is very suited for diagnosis of disorders in the pediatric hip such as Perthes disease. Perthes disease is easily differentiated from transient synovitis in a patient with an irritable hip. In Perthes disease, a decreased signal intensity in epiphyseal bone marrow, identical to changes found in osteonecrosis in the adult, are present in an early stage (Fig.7). An accompanying joint effusion is also frequently found. In transient synovitis, joint effusion with a normal epiphysis is seen.

The three dimensional display of necrotic bone in Perthes disease may become important in staging and may thus facilitate planning and timing of surgical procedures. For this purpose a combination of sagittal and coronal views are needed.

Containment of the femoral head and development of the necrotic area following surgical therapy can be evaluated with MRI.

Prognostic MRI factors, similar to prognostic radiographic factors (Caterell classification) are not yet known, but will be evaluated in the near future.

MUSCULOSKELETAL TUMORS

Historically, a mutilating surgical procedure has been the most effective method of treating the majority of primary malignant musculoskeletal tumors. The efficacy of recently introduced chemotherapeutic agents coupled with advances in radiation therapy and surgical techniques, has fostered an interest in more conservative surgery in combination with reconstructive procedures for restoring function.

Successful treatment of patients with musculoskeletal tumors depends to a large extent on meticulous pretreatment staging.

In a prospective study of 65 patients MRI, CT, Tc-99m MDP scintigraphy and angiography were correlated with of pathological examination of the resected specimens. The accuracy of MRI is significantly higher than the accuracy of CT, Tc-99m MDP scintigraphy and angiography in determining the intra- and extraosseous tumor extension (2,3,6). MRI is the only modality which can visualize all important anatomical structures in relation with

pathology in one examination (Fig.8).
   T1 weighted images in the sagittal or coronal plane are used to define
intra-medullary extension. T2 weighted images in the transverse plane are
used to visualize cortical involvement and soft tissue extension (Fig.9).
Additional longitudinal views are frequently used to demonstrate the relationship with joints.
   A specific histologic diagnosis is rarely made with the aid of MRI (4)
because most tumors have a typical low signal intensity on T1 and a high
signal intensity on T2 weighted images (Fig.9). Some tumors have however a
specific appearance on MRI (4):

- osteosclerotic osteosarcoma has a very low signal intensity, even on T2
weighted images.
- Teleangiectatic osteosarcoma, aneurysmal bone cyst and highly vascular
tumors such as angiosarcoma have a relatively high signal intensity on T1
weighted images (Fig.10) (1). Highly vascular lesions are often characterized by flow void areas (Fig.11).
- Cartilage has a relatively high signal intensity on T1 and especially T2
weighted images. The cartilage tumor often has a characteristic polyglo-
bular appearance (Fig.12).
- Pigmented villonodular synovitis has a very low signal intensity on T1
and T2 weighted images because of the paramagnetic effect of the high iron
concentration present in these disorders (Fig.13).
The overall specificity remains poor and MRI cannot be used to differentiate benign from malignant tumors.
The use of Gd-DTPA may sometimes increase specificity (4). Enhancement
patterns facilitate identification of viable and necrotic tumor tissue,
edema, hematoma and non enhancing cartilage (Fig.14). In cartilage tumors
a typical peripheral enhancement pattern is found (Fig.12). The central
cartilage containing part does not enhance. This pattern must be differentiated from tumors with necrosis. A second advantage of Gd-DTPA enhanced short SE sequences is that they can replace the more time consuming T2
weighted SE sequences.
   Chemical shift images are sometimes useful to enhance contrast between
tumor and normal bone marrow (Fig.15).
   MRI is able to monitor the effect of chemotherapy. Change of tumor volume and signal intensities can be evaluated. A decrease (dehydration,
fibrosis, calcification) or an increase (necrosis) of signal intensity on
T2 weighted images indicates a satisfactory response. A stable signal intensity indicates an unsatisfactory response.

OSTEOMYELITIS
   Osteomyelitis has an aspecific low signal intensity on T1 weighted images and a high signal intensity on T2 weighted images (Fig.4,16) (5). The
signal intensity is thus identical to tumor. Only the relatively indistinct border of inflammatory tissue may sometimes be differentiated from
the relatively distinct margin of neoplasm.
   MRI may be useful in the diagnosis of osteomyelitis if the Tc-99m MDP
scan is equivocal, for instance when preexistent disease such as fracture,
infarction, or Gaucher's disease is present (Fig.4) (1).
   MRI is extremely sensitive and specific in the diagnosis of spondylitis
(1,13). MRI may thus be used to diagnose soft tissue infection, spondylitis, or degenerative disc disease (Fig.17,18).

206

CONCLUSION
   After only a few years of clinical research, MRI of the musculoskeletal
system is a clinical reality. In our institution MRI is routinely used in
the diagnostic work-up of patients with musculoskeletal tumors. MRI is
frequently used in patients with osteomyelitis, spondylitis, osteonecrosis
and bone marrow disorders. The definite place of MRI in relation to other
diagnostic procedures is not yet settled, but its potential is great, and
it is becoming one of the most important diagnostic procedures in musculoskeletal disease (7).

Acknowledgements: Gd-DTPA was kindly supplied by Schering AG. The present
study was partly subsidized by the Dutch Cancer Foundation (IKW grant
8589). Figure 2 was reprinted with permission from reference 14. Figures
1,6,7 are reprinted with permission from reference 1. Figures 5 and 11 are
reprinted with permission from reference 7.

REFERENCES
1 Bloem J.L., Taminiau A.H.M., Kieft G.J., et al.: MRI van het Steun- en
   Bewegingsapparaat. NTVG 1987; 30: 1311-1316.

2 Bloem J.L., Falke T.H.M., Taminiau A.H.M., et al: MRI of Primary Malignant Bone Tumors. Radiographics 1985; 5: 853-886.

3 Bloem J.L., Bluemm R.G., Taminiau A.H.M., et al: MRI of Primary Malignant Bone Tumors, Radiographics 1987; 7, 3: 425-445.

4 Bloem J.L., Bluemm R.G., Taminiau A.H.M., et al: MRI of Primary Malignant Musculoskeletal Tumors. In: Nuclear Magnetic Resonance Imaging;
   editor C.L. Partain, in press.

5 Bloem J.L, Falke T.H.M., Doornbos J.: Osteomyelitis in Children: Detection by MRI. Radiology 1984; 153: 263.

6 Bloem J.L., Taminiau A.H.M., Eulderink F., et al.: The impact of MRI is
   staging musculoskeletal tumors, a prospective study of 65 patients.
   Society of Magnetic Resonance in Medicine. Abstract book 1987, in
   press.

7 Bloem J.L., Taminiau A.H.M., Kieft G.J., et al.: MRI and CT in orthopedics. In Documed Proceedings Elsevier 1987, in press.

8. Bluemm R.G., Falke T.H.M., Ziedses des Plantes Jr T.H.M., Steiner R.M.:
   Early Legg-Perthes disease (ischemic necrosis of the femoral head) demonstrated by magnetic resonance imaging. Skeletal Radiol 1985; 14:
   98-98.

9. Lamir A., Hadar H., Cohen I., et al: Gaucher disease: assessment with
   MR imaging. Radiology 1986; 161: 239.

10. Mckinstry C.S., Steiner R.E., Young A.T., et al: Bone marrow in leu-
    kaemia and aplastic anemia: MR imaging before, during and after treat-
    ment. Radiology 1987; 162: 701-707.

11. Mitchell D.G., Rao V.M., Dalinka M.K., et al: Femoral Head avascular
    necrosis: correlation of MR imaging, radiographic staging, radionuclide
    imaging and clinical findings. Radiology 1987; 162: 709-715

12. Mitchell M.D., Kundel H.L., Steinberg M.E., et al: Avascular Necrosis
    of the Hip: Comparison of MR, CT and Scintigraphy. AJR 1986; 147:
    67-71.

13. De Roos A., Van Persijn van Meerten E.L., Bloem J.L., et al: MRI of
    Tuberculous Spondylitis. AJR 1986; 146: 79-82.

14. Tjon A Tham R.T.O, Bloem J.L., Falke T.H.M., et al: MRI in Paget's Dis-
    ease of the Skull. AJNR 1985; 6: 879-881.

208

FIGURE 1   Acute lymphatic leukaemia.
            Coronal view (TR 550, TR 30).
            The left femoral epiphysis has a normal high signal intensity.
            The decreased signal intensity seen in the spine, pelvis,
            right epiphysis and both femur metaphyses represents diffuse
            leukaemic infiltration.

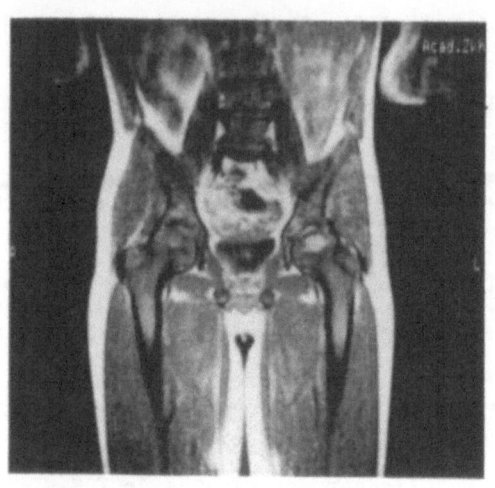

FIGURE 2   Paget's disease.
            Sagittal view (TR 1000, TE 50), 0.15 T.
            Thickening of diploic space with corresponding thinning of
            inner and outer tables is seen. The irregular margin of the
            frontal lobe is caused by compression of the thickened calva-
            ria.

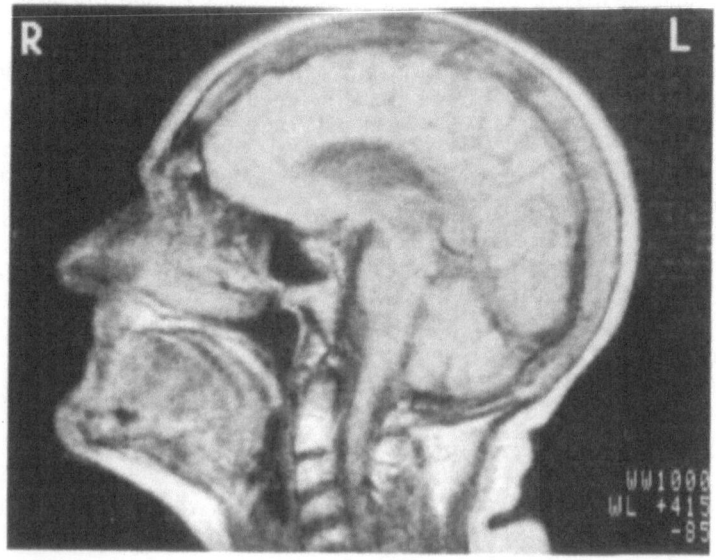

FIGURE 3   Paget's disease of the tibia.
a) Sagittal view (TR 550, TE 30).
The cortex is thickened at at the site of the anterior tubercle. Abnormal cortex has an intermediate signal intensity. Bone marrow is completely normal.
b) Transverse view (TR 2000, TE 50).
Intermediate signal intensity of Paget's disease in the anterior cortex is easily differentiated from normal cortex and normal bone marrow.
At histological examination Paget's disease was found.

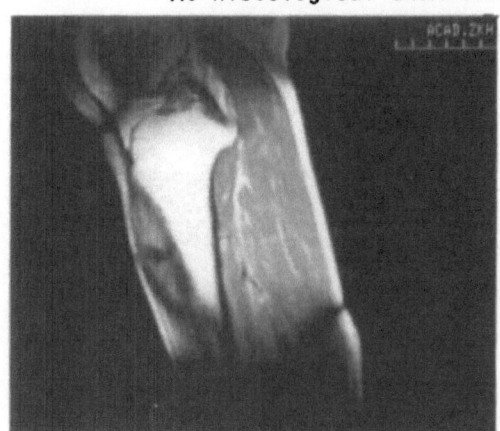 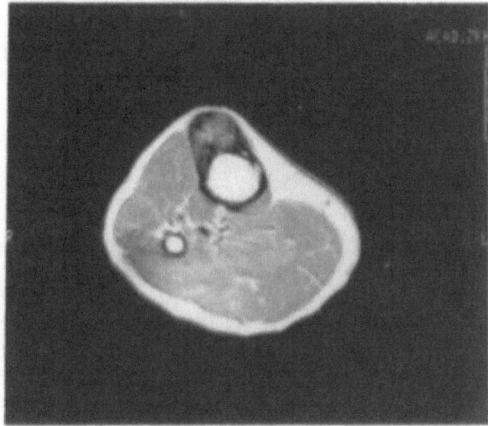

FIGURE 4   Osteomyelitis complicating Gaucher's disease.
a) Coronal view (TR 550, TE 30).
The low signal intensity of bone marrow in the left femur combined with the flask deformity is compatible with Gaucher's disease.
b) Coronal view (TR 1500, TE 100).
The high signal intensity is atypical for Gaucher's disease but is in accordance with osteomyelitis, complicating Gaucher's disease. The patient was successfully treated with antibiotics following culture.

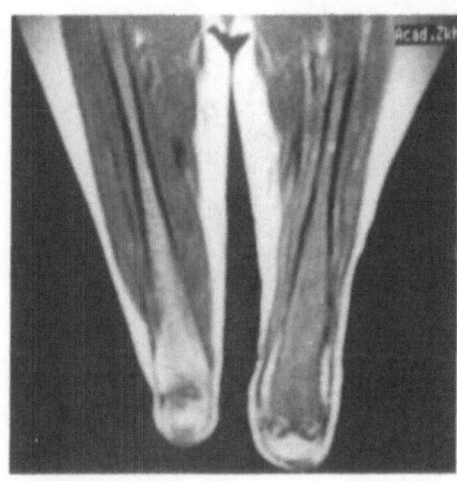 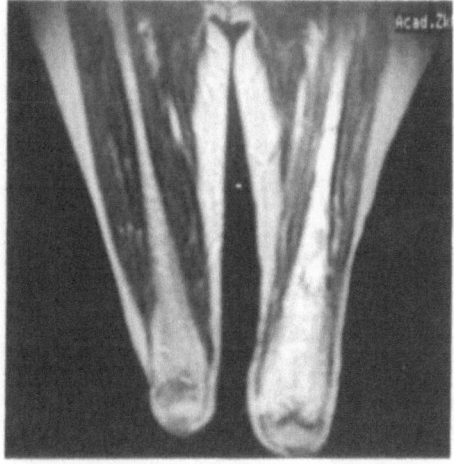

FIGURE 5   Transient ischemic osteoporosis (TIA).
a) Coronal view (TR 550, TE 30).
This 15-year old male complained of pain in the left hip. On
this T1 weighted image a decreased signal intensity is easily
appreciated in the left proximal femur.
b) Transverse view (TR 2400, TE 100).
The lesion has an increased signal intensity on this T2
weighted image.
At histological examination, reactive changes were found,
culture was negative. A diagnosis of TIA was made and the patient was not treated.
c) Coronal view (TR 550, TE 30).
Three months after Fig.5a, the signal intensity is now
completely normal. The patient at this time did not have any
complaints.

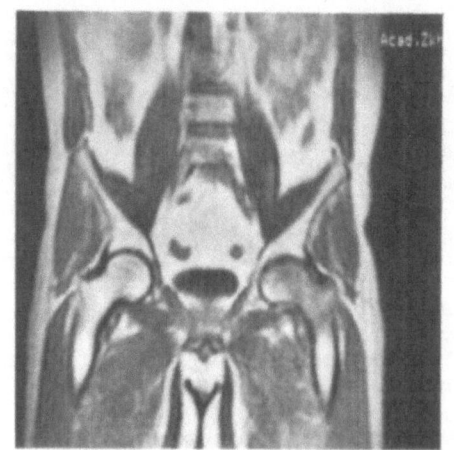
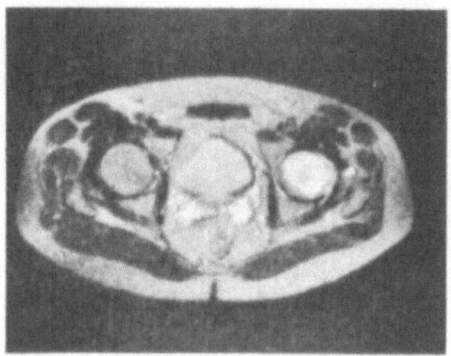

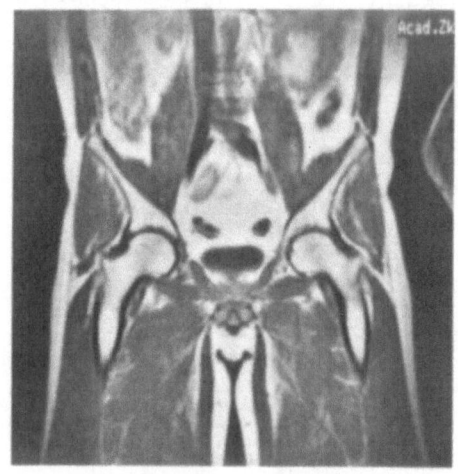

FIGURE 6 Osteonecrosis.
　　　a) Coronal view (TR 550, TE 30).
　　　　This patient was suspected of having left sided osteonecrosis.
　　　　Tc-99 m MDP scintigraphy demonstrated increased uptake on the
　　　　left side. The right hip was normal. On MRI a low signal in-
　　　　tensity area is seen in the left epi-metaphyseal region. This
　　　　in accordance with osteonecrosis. On the asymptomatic right
　　　　side, a band-like decreased signal intensity region can be
　　　　depicted, this is is also in accordance with osteonecrosis.
　　　b) Coronal view (TR 550, TE 30).
　　　　Three months later, the patient complained of pain in the
　　　　left and right hip. Progression of both necrotic regions is
　　　　easily appreciated. Tc-99m MDP scintigraphy showed an increa-
　　　　sed uptake in both hips at this time.

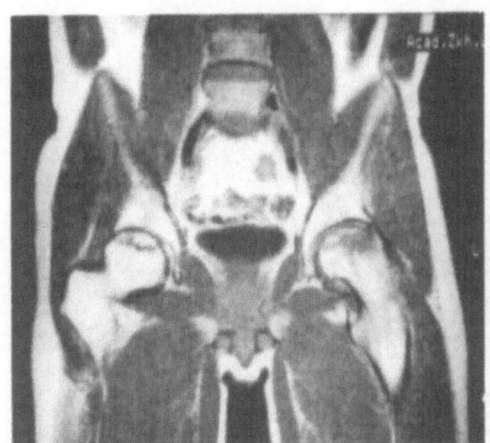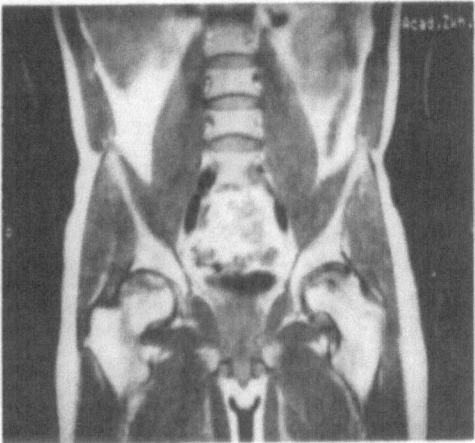

FIGURE 7 Perthes disease.
　　　A decreased signal intensity located in the left epiphysis
　　　represents the aréa of necrosis.

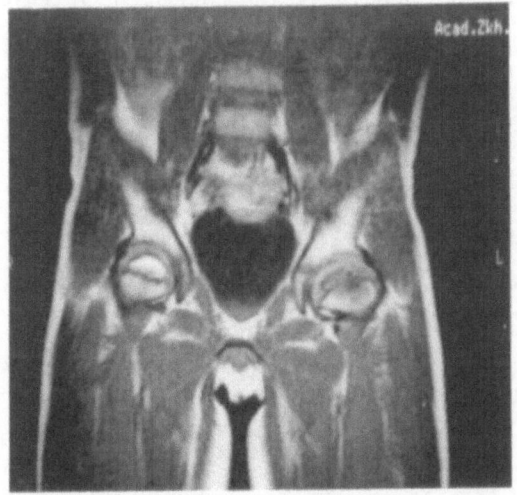

FIGURE 8 Juxtacortical osteosarcoma.
  a) Sagittal view (TR 550, TE 30).
     The tumor has a relative low signal intensity. Bone marrow infiltration and displacement of femoral artery re depicted.
  b) Transverse view (TR 2000, TE 50).
     Tumor has a intermediate signal intensity. The intimate contact between neurovascular bundle (arrows) and tumor is easily appreciated. There is no encasement. This patient was treated with local resection.

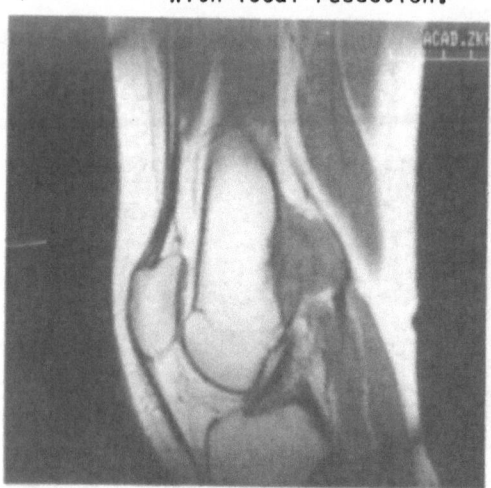 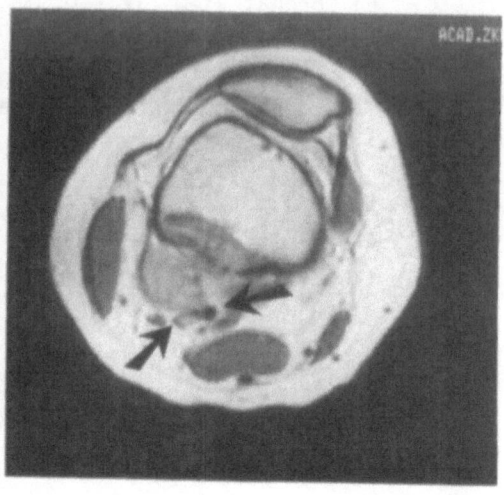

FIGURE 9 Ewing sarcoma of the femur.
  a) Coronal view (TR 550, TE 30).
     High contrast between the low signal intensity of tumor and high signal intensity of normal bone marrow allows accurate intramedullary staging.
  b) Transverse view (TR 2000, TE 50).
     The high signal intensity of tumor allows accurate staging of soft tissue extension. Tumor infiltrates medial vastus compartment. The neurovascular bundle is free of tumor at this level.
     The cortex is infiltrated circumferentially (compare the black line of normal cortical bone on the left side).

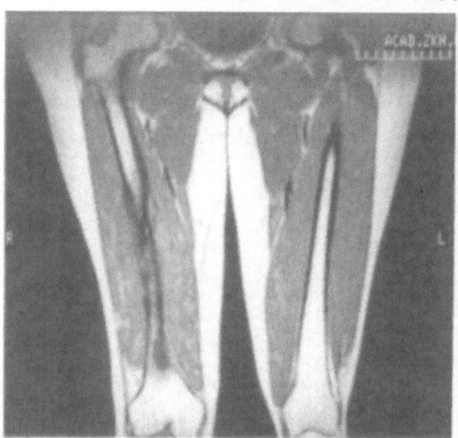 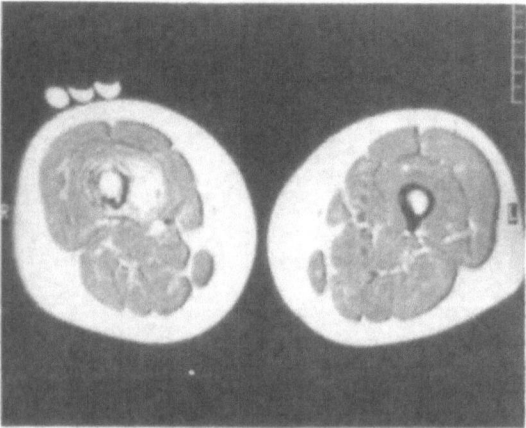

FIGUUR 10 Teleangiectatic osteosarcoma.
Sagittal view (TR 550, TE 30).
The central part of the tumor has, in contrast to the major
tumor area, an increased signal intensity on this T1 weighted
image.
This indicates hemorrhage and is compatible with diagnosis of
teleangiectatic osteosarcoma.

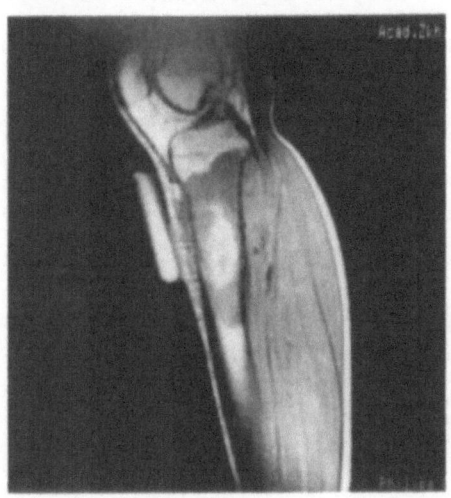

FIGURE 11 Arterio-venous malformation, two contiguous sections sagittal
(TR 550, TE 30).
The AV malformation as well as the feeding and draining vessels are seen as black structures because of rapid flow. Extensive intramedullary as well as soft tissue involvement is
easily appreciated.

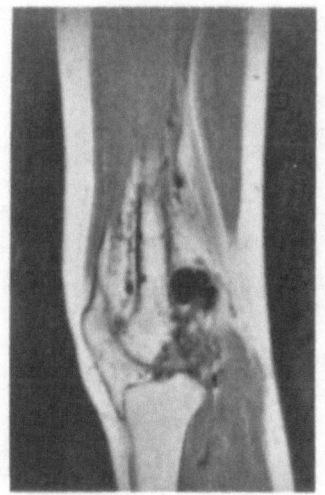 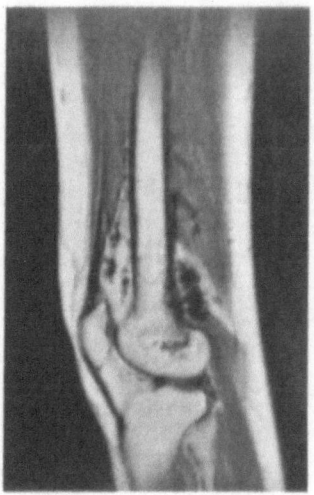

FIGURE 12 Chondrosarcoma of the spine.
a) Coronal view (TR 2000, TE 100).
The lobulated tumor has a high signal intensity. This is characteristic for a non-calcified cartilage tumor.
b) Coronal view (TR 550, TE 30).
The lobulated tumor has a low signal intensity. This is atypical for chondrosarcoma.
c) Coronal view (TR 550, TE 30) 5 minutes following I.V. administration of Gd-DTPA.
The ring enhancement is typical for cartilage containing tumors.

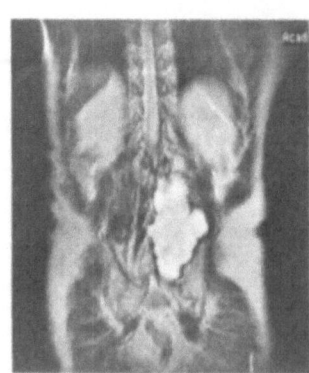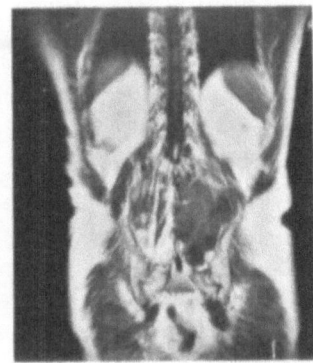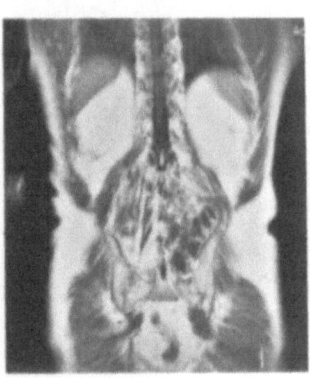

FIGURE 13 Pigmented villonodular synovitis.
a) Sagittal view (TR 550, TE 30).
The lobulad lesion is located on the posterior side of the
joint and encroaches upon the talus. The signal intensity is
low.
b) Sagittal view (TR 2000, TE 100).
On this heavily T2 weighted image, the signal intensity is
persistently low because of a short T2 relaxation time.

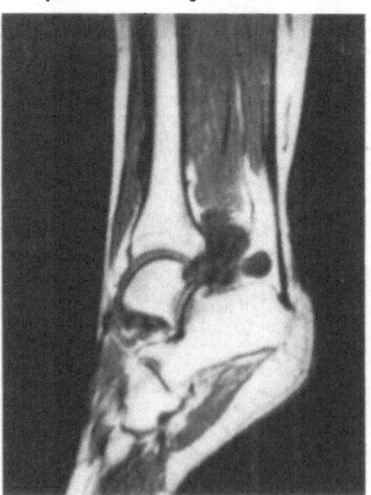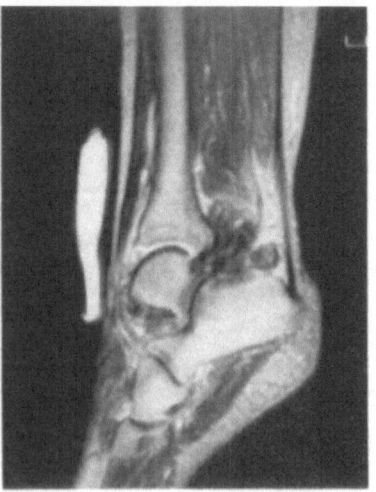

FIGURE 14 Synovial sarcoma of the right hip.
  a) Coronal view (TR 550, TE 30).
     The synovia sarcoma infiltrates the femur. Note high contrast
     between the low signal intensity of tumor and high signal in-
     tensity of normal bone marrow.
  b) Transverse view (TR 550, TE 30).
     Contrast between tumor and muscular tissue is poor on this T1
     weighted image because signal intensities of these two struc-
     tures are similar.
  c) Transverse view (TR 2000, TE 100).
     The tumor is, on this T2 weighted image, seen as a high signal
     intensity area. Contrast between tumor and normal muscular
     tissue is high.
  d) Gd-DTPA enhanced coronal view (TR 550, TE 30).
     Tumor enhancement of tumor results via shortening of the T2
     relaxation time, in an increased signal intensity on this
     short SE sequences. Note the high signal intensity in the
     bladder caused by accumulation of Gd-DTPA which is excreted by
     the kidneys.

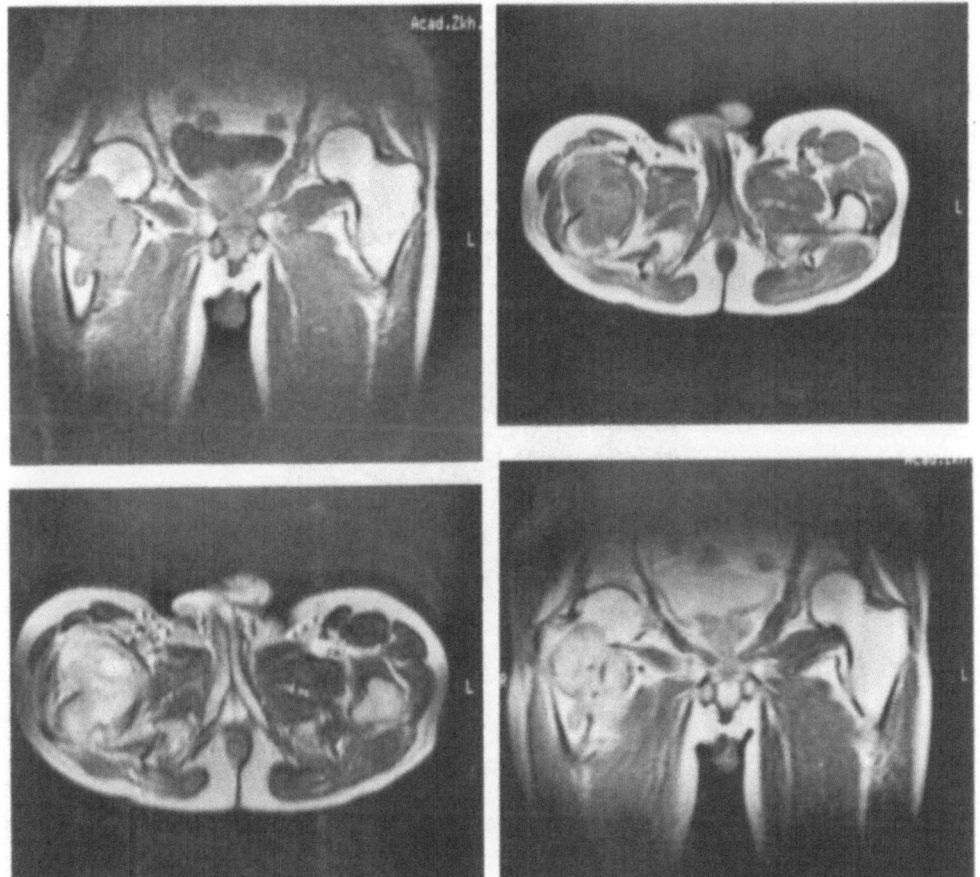

216

FIGURE 15 Chondroblastoma of the tibia.
          a) Coronal view (TR 1000, TE 30).
             Contrast between the tumor and surrounding bone marrow is
             rather poor.
          b) Coronal view, water image. The tumor has a high signal inten-
             sity because of its high water content.
          c) Coronal view, fat image. The tumor contains little fat and is
             therefore represented by a low signal intensity area.

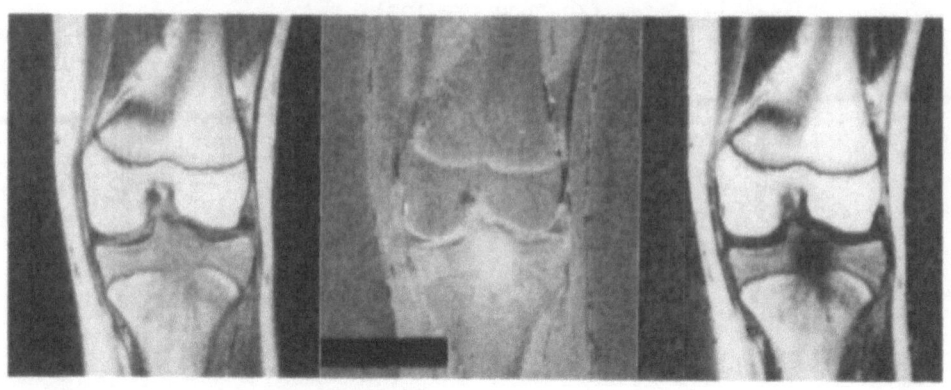

FIGUUR 16 Chronic osteomyelitis.
          Sagittal view (TR 2000, TE 100).
          Active inflammatory tissue is represented by high signal in-
          tensity in the femur, joint and soft tissues.

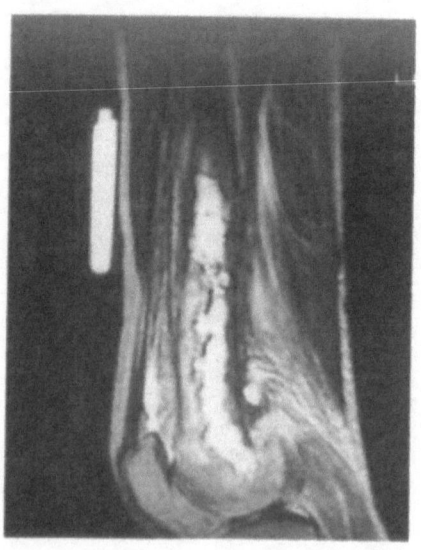

FIGUUR 17 Soft tissue infection (corynebacterium). This patient with
claustrofobia was examined in the prone position. Images were
made with one excitation.
a) Coronal view (TR 2000, TE 50).
Inflammatory tissue is represented by the paravertebral high
signal intensity (arrows).
b) Sagittal view (TR 2000, TE 100).
Bone scintigraphy suggested spondylitis, but this sagittal
view exhibits normal intervertebral discs and   therefore
excludes spondylitis.

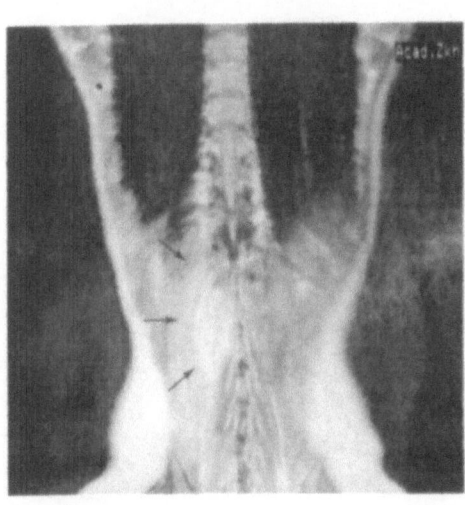 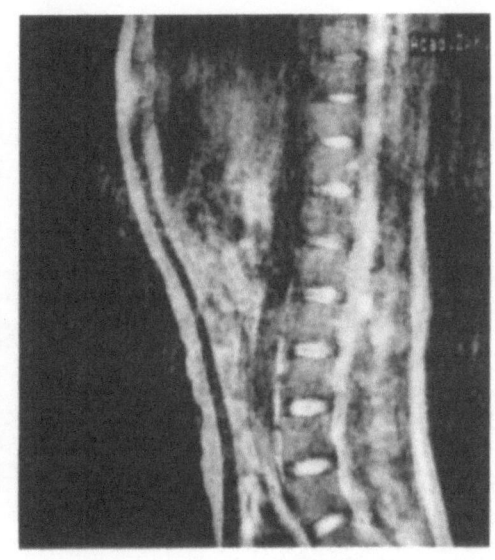

FIGURE 18 Schmorl node in a 10-year old child.
a) This patient with pain in the lumbar spine displayed an
increased uptake of Tc-99m MDP at the L IV-V level. Clinically
a tumor was expected.
b) Sagittal view (TR 2000, TE 100).
The intervertebral disc LIV-V protrudes into the spongiosa of
LIV and LV. No tumor was present.

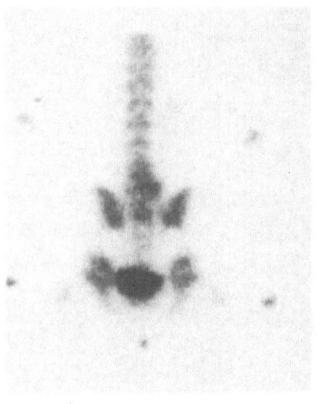 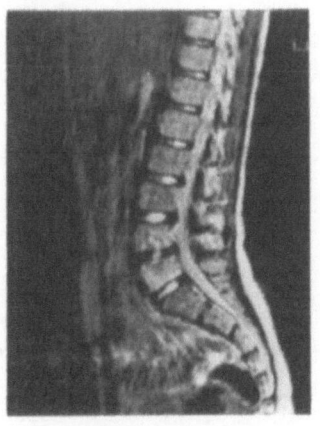

MRI OF ADULT AND PEDIATRIC JOINT DISEASE

J.L. BLOEM, G.J. KIEFT, C.F.M. BOS, P.M. ROZING

INTRODUCTION
   Many research institutions have explored the potential of MRI in imaging
normal structures and pathologic alterations in and around the joints
(1,4,5,9). MRI is in this field competing with procedures such a conventional roentgenograms, ultrasound, CT, arthrography, computerized arthro-
tomography and arthroscopy. Advantages of MRI in this perspective are its
direct visualization of soft tissue structures in multiple planes with
superior contrast resolution and its non-invasive character. In addition
MRI is easy to perform. As experience accumulates it appears that acces to
information provided by MRI is easy both to radiologists and clinicians.
   This chapter presents some characteristic MR images and discusses the
potential of MRI. The presented images were made with a 0.5 T Philips Gyroscan. Different anatomically tailored surface coils were used. Relative
T1 (550/30) and T2 weighted (2000-50/100) spin echo images were made.

Traumatic disorders
   MRI is very sensitive in visualizing in a non-invasive way abnormalities
in the acutely traumatized joint. A joint effusion often facilitates evaluation of the interior of the joint.
   In the knee joint rupture of collateral and cruciate ligaments as well
as meniscal tear can be accurately visualized (Fig.1,2) (8,10,11,13,14).
The meniscus including the posterior horn is easily visualized over its
entire length when coronal and sagittal images are made. The negative
predictive value for meniscal tear is reported to be almost 100% (11). The
posterior cruciate ligament is easily visualized in the sagittal plane.
The anterior cruciate ligament is thinner and is because of its obliquely
orientated course best visualized with a combination of sagittal and
oblique sagittal (10-20°) views. MRI is in contrast to arthrography able
to demonstrate a rupture of the ligaments, even when the synovial covering
of the cruciate ligaments is intact. A traumatized ligament is characterized by an increased signal intensity and a indistinct margin of the ligament. A severely traumatized ligament is often not directly visualized.
Because a diagnosis of ruptured cruciate ligament is made by virtue of its
absence in combination with secondary changes (Fig.2), the area of the
ligament has to be evaluated in at least two planes. Edema and haematoma
are seen as a mass of increased signal intensity.
The sensitivity for rupture of the cruciate ligaments is 96% (14).
   In the traumatized shoulder, tear or entrapment of the biceps tendon
stripping of the anterior capsule as well as tear of the labrum (cartila-
genous Bankart lesion) and osseous lesions (osseous Bankart and Hill-Sachs
lesions) can be visualized in one noninvasive examination without using
intraarticular contrast agents (Fig.3) (7). The optimal imaging planes are
the transverse plane and a longitudinal plane perpendicular to the glenoid
(6). In this stage partial rotator cuff tears or those without diastasis
are difficult to visualize with MRI.
   Ruptured ligaments and muscles around other joints are also easily
appreciated (Fig.4,5).

Chronic disorders
   In impingement syndrome of the shoulder, the archictecture of the cora-

coacromial arc and its relationship to the rotator cuff and humeral head can be evaluated. The impingement of the coracoacromial arc and the ensuing degeneration and inflammation of the tendon and subsequent atrophy of the supraspinatus muscle are best demonstrated on longitudinal views, perpendicular to the glenoid (Fig.6,7) (7).

Effects of arthritis such as effusion, synovial inflammation and destruction of cartilage, capsule and tendons can be depicted in a non-invasive way with MRI before osseous destruction is seen on conventional roentgenograms (Fig.8).

The inflammatory tissue found in rheumatoid arthritis and the effect of C1-C2 dislocation on the spinal cord and brain stem can be directly visualized not only in the neutral position but also in flexion and extension (12).

Tumors and tumor-like lesions can be detected with high sensitivity. MRI visualizes joint disorders in any desired imaging plane with high contrast, and therefore facilitates planning of surgical procedures (Fig.9,10) (2).

<u>Congenital hip dysplasia</u>
Congenital dislocation of the hip is preferably treated by conservative means. If however conservative treatment fails, surgical treatment has to be considered. Diagnostic procedures are needed to select the appropriate form of therapy. Information about obstructing factors is needed. In time these obstructions may become adaptive and may not be overcome by conservative treatment. Up until now arthrography was the most accurate way to demonstrate obstructing factors. The indications for MRI are similar to those for arthrography.

MRI may be used in complicated cases: when reduction fails, when redislocation occurs and when the presence of a concentric reduction is questioned. MRI has several advantages over arthrography: MRI is noninvasive and has thus no risk of infection, it does not use ionizing radiation and usually can be performed without anesthesia. In our experience 85-90% of patients in this age group can be examined with mild sedation only.

Impeding structures such as the limbus, the ligamentum teres and pulvinar can be identified with MRI (Fig.11,12). Hypertrophy of the acetabular cartilage, joint effusion and muscular athrophy are all visualized. Incongruity of the hip and its cause are thus easily detected.

These findings may help in selecting the appropriate form of conservative or surgical therapy. In addition the response to therapy and development of the hip can be closely monitored (3).

CONCLUSION
The potential of MRI to diagnose joint disorders is high. A high signal-to-noise ratio is needed to obtain the necessary anatomical resolution. The potential of MRI is especially high in systems with a field strength of 1-2 T (9). Small joints such as the temperomandibular joint and the wrist can be evaluated with high field systems (4,14). High quality surface coils however allow MRI of joint disease at superconductive MRI units with a field strenght of 0.5 T.

Comparitive studies are needed to determine the place of MRI between the existing diagnostic modalities. MRI may have a place in diagnosis of the acutely traumatized joint because it is a non-invasive alternative to arthroscopy or arthrotomy in a situation in which clinical examination is often unreliable. Diagnosis of impingement syndrome and evaluation of rheumatoid arthritis in the cervical spine and staging of congenital hip dysplasia may have a major impact on patient management.

REFERENCES
1. Beltran J., Noto A.M., Mosure J.C., et al.: The knee: surface coil MR imaging at 1.5 T. Radiology 1986; 159: 747-751.

2. Bloem J.L., Taminiau A.H.M, Bos C.F.A., et al.: MRI and CT in orthopedics. In Documed Proceedings Elseviers 1987, in press.

3. Bos C.F.M., Bloem J.L., Obermann W.R., et al.: MRI in congenital dislocation of the hip. Journal of Bone and Joint Surgery 1987; B: in press.

4. Harms S.E., Wick R.M.,: Magnetic resonance imaging of the temporomandibular joint. Radiographics 1987; 7(3): 521-542.

5. Hajek P.C., Baker L.L., Sartoris D.J., et al.: MR arthrography: anatomic pathologic investigation. Radiology 1987; 163: 141-147.

6. Kieft G.J., Bloem, J.L., Obermann, W.R., et al.: Normal shoulder : MR imaging. Radiology 1986; 159: 741-745.

7. Kieft G.J., Sartoris D.J., Bloem J.L., et al.: MRI of glenohumeral joint disease. Skeletal Radiology 1987; 16: 285-290.

8. Manco L.G., Lozman J., Coleman M.D.: noninvasive evaluation of knee meniscal tears: preliminary comparison of MR imaging and CT. Radiology 1987; 163: 727-730.

9. Middleton W.D., Macrander S., Lawson T.L., et al.: High resolution surface coil magnetic resonance imaging of the joints: anatomic correlation. Radiographics 1987; 7(4): 645-683.

10. Reichner M.A., Hartzman S., Bassett L.W., et al.: MR imaging of the knee. Part I Traumatic Disorders. Radiology 1987; 547-551.

11. Reicher M.A., Hartzman S., Duckwiler G.R.: Meniscal injuries: detection using MR imaging. Radiology 1986; 159: 753-757.

12. Reynolds H., Carter S.W., Murtagh F.R., Rechtime G.R.: Cervical rheumatoid arthritis: value of flexion and extension views in imaging. Radiology 1987; 164: 215-218.

13. Stoller D.W., Martin C., Cruess III J.V., et al.: Meniscal Tears: pathologic correlation with MR imaging.

14. Turner D.A., Prodromos C.L., Petasnick J.P., et al.: Acute Injury of the ligaments of the knee: magnetic resonance evaluation. Radiology 1985; 154: 717-723.

15. Weiss K.L., Beltran J., Shaman O.M., Stilla R.F., Levey M. High field MR surface coil imaging of the hand and wrist: Part II. Pathologic correlations and clinical relevance. Radiology 1986; 160: 147-152.

FIGURE 1a) Tear in the medial meniscus.
Sagittal view (TR 550, TE 30).
The increased signal intensity line represents a tear in the
posterior horn of the lateral meniscus (arrow).
1b) Coronal view (TR 550, TE 30).
The tear extends into the medial zone of the lateral meniscus
(arrow).

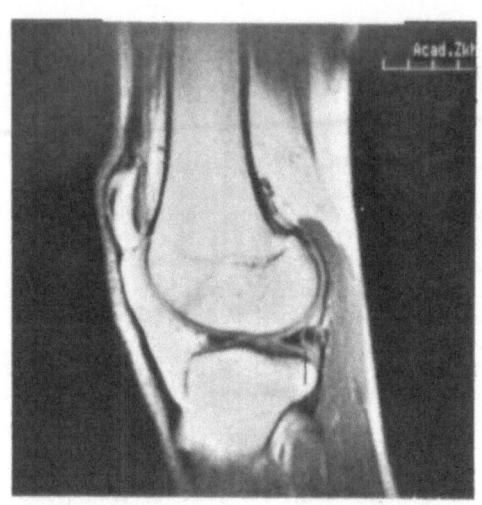

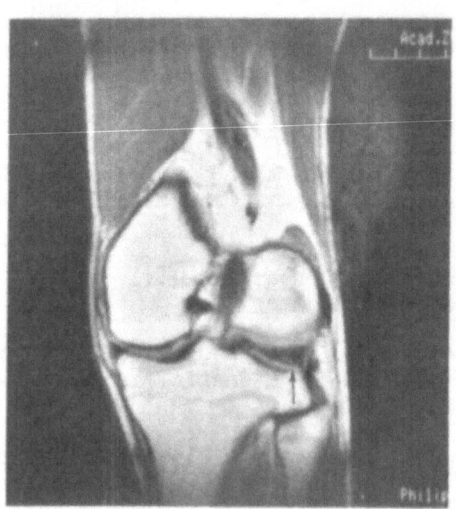

FIGURE 2   Acutely traumatized knee.
   a) Sagittal view (TR 550, TE 30).
      Joint effusion is seen anterior to the medial condyle. The
      increased signal intensity line in the posterior horn of the
      medial meniscus represents a tear which was also seen at
      arthrography (arrow).
   b) Sagittal view (TR 550, TE 30).
      More medial than 2a, the joint effusion is now clearly visi-
      ble. The normal posterior cruciate ligament is visualized.
   c) Sagittal view (TR 550, TE 30).
      The anterior cruciate ligament cannot be identified and is
      replaced by an indistinct soft tissue mass representing edema
      and hematoma. The ruptured anterior cruciate ligament was
      found at surgery but was not detected by arthrography,
      arthroscopy and clinical examination under anesthesia.

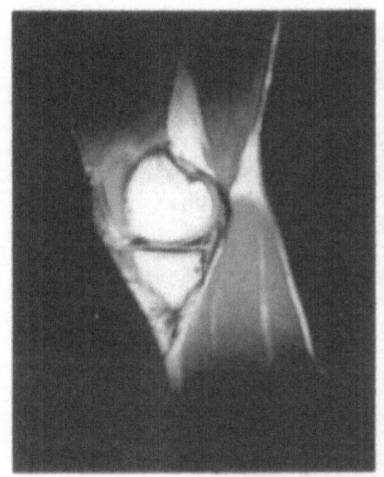 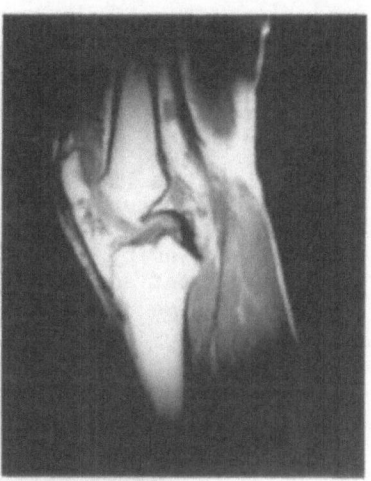

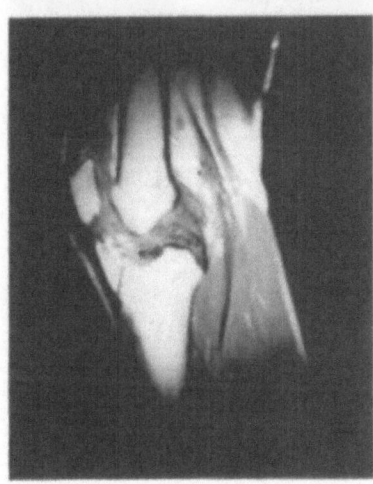

FIGURE 3   Anterior glenohumeral dislocation, five days following reduc-
             tion.
        a) Transverse view (TR 1500, TE 30).
           In addition to joint effusion, stripping (arrow) of the cap-
           sule from the anterior aspect of the glenoid can be depicted.
        b) Longitudinal view, perpendicular to the glenoid.
           (TR 1500, TE 50).
           The torn fragment of the labrum is demonstrated, caudal to the
           glenoid (arrow).

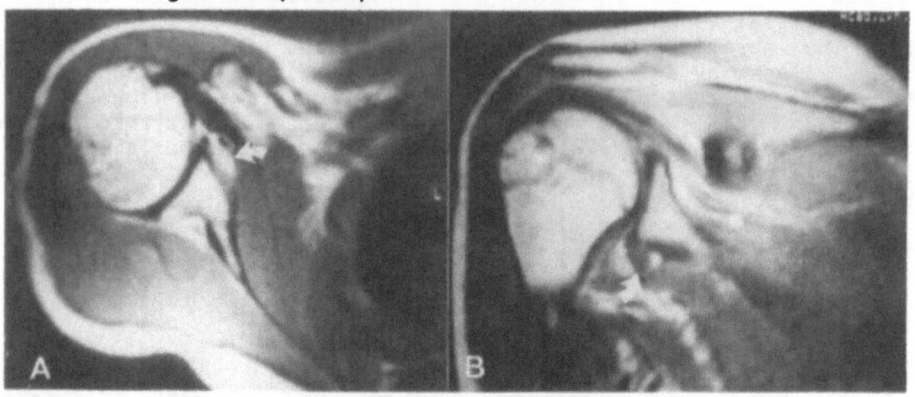

FIGURE 4   Complete rupture of the achilles tendon.
             Sagittal view (TR 600, TE 30).
             A discontinuity of the achilles tendon is clearly visualized.
             Hematoma and edema is seen as an increased signal intensity
             area between calcaneus and tendon.

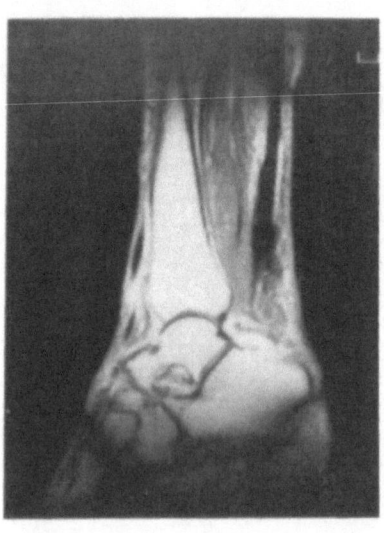

FIGURE 5   Incomplete rupture of the Achilles Tendon.
a) Sagittal view (TR 550, TE 30).
The partially ruptured Achilles tendon is thickened and has areas of increased signal intensity. The continuity is preserved.
b) Transverse view (TR 550, TE 30).
The increased signal intensity caused by hemorrhage is clearly demonstrated in the thickened tendon.

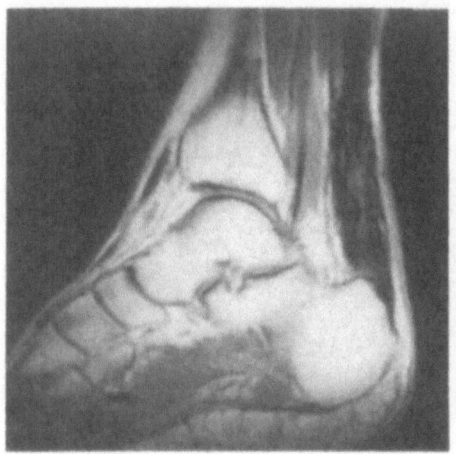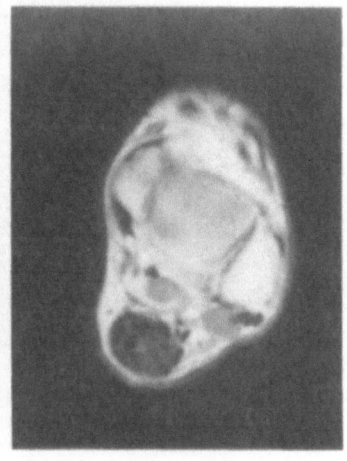

FIGURE 6   Impingement syndrome.
Oblique longitudinal view, perpendicular to the glenoid.
(TR 600, TE 30).
Osseous impingement at the level of the acromioclavicular joint can be depicted.
The tendon of the supraspinatus muscle has an increased signal intensity compatible with tendinitis (arrow).

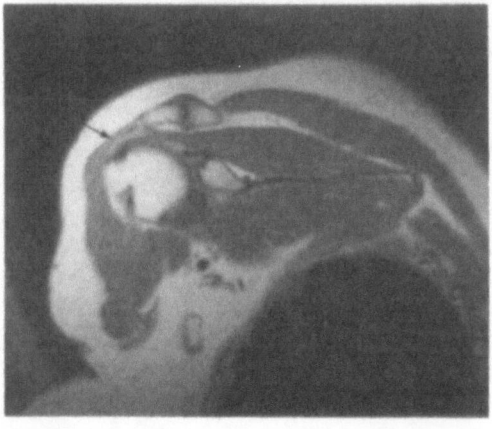

FIGURE 7 Clinical impingement syndrome. Oblique longitudinal view perpendicular to the glenoid.
(TR 600, TE 30).
The thinned supraspinatus muscle displays an increased signal intensity at the (juxta) tendinous part of the supraspinatus muscle (arrow). This allows a diagnosis of tendinitis to be made.

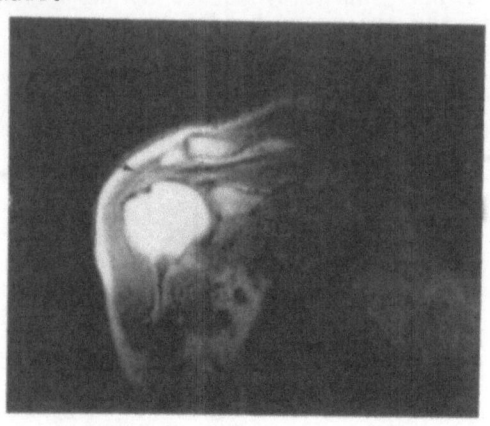

FIGURE 8 Rheumatoid arthritis.
Transverse view (TR 1050, TE 50).
The soft tissue which exhibits an increased signal intensity represents a large synovial cyst (arrow).
A concomittant joint effusion is present.

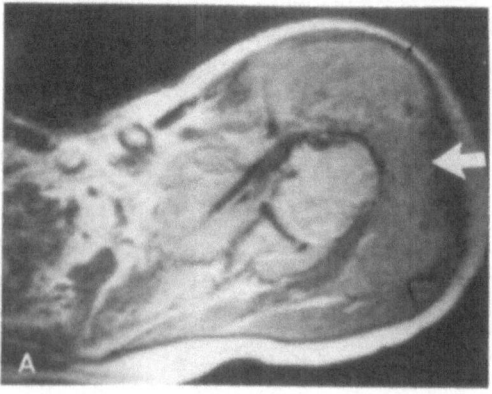

FIGURE 9   Giant cell tumor.
            Sagittal view (TR 550, TE 30).
            The posterior cruciate ligament is easily identified and in-
            serts in the tumor.

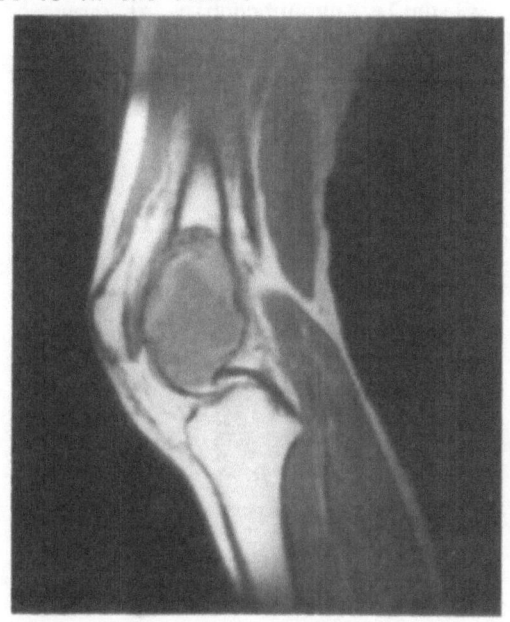

FIGURE 10 Synovial chondromatosis.
         a) Sagittal view (TR 1650, TE 50).
            On this relatively T2 weighted image, the signal intensity of
            non-calcified cartilage is high.
         b) Coronal view (TR 300, TE 30).
            The persistence of high signal intensity on this relatively T1
            weighted image is consistent with the presence of non-calci-
            fied cartilage.

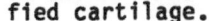

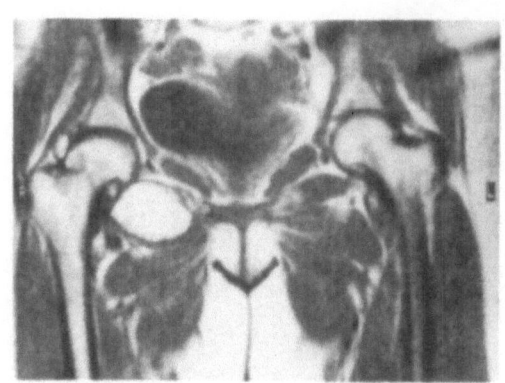

228

FIGURE 11 Congenital hip dysplasia without interposition of the limbus.
Coronal view (TR 550, TE 30).
The left femur is anteriorly displaced. The limbus is everted
and does not block the entrance to the acetabulum (arrow). The
pulvinar is slightly hypertrophic as compared to the right
side. Note a normal limbus on the right side.

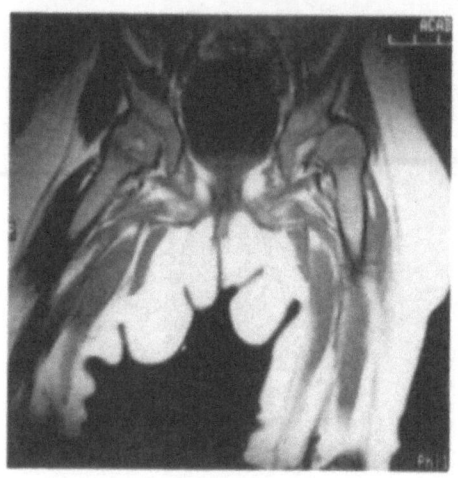

FIGURE 12 Congenital hip dysplasia with limbus interposition.
Coronal view (TR 550, TE 30).
The left hip is displaced superiorly. The entrance to the
acetabulum is blocked by the inverted limbus (arrow).

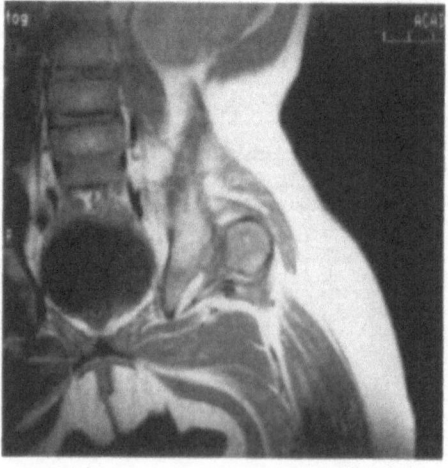

CLINICAL RELEVANCE OF MRI IN THE EVALUATION OF MUSKULOSKELETAL DISEASE

A.H.M. TAMINIAU
C.F.A. BOS ·

In the evaluation of musculoskeletal disease conventional radiographs and techniques such as conventional tomography and computed tomography will deliver the information needed in most cases.

If additional information concerning disease processes of joints, bone marrow, soft tissues and vascular structures is required, Magnetic Resonance Imaging (MRI) can be very useful.
MRI is especially helpful in the visualization of these structures, and the relation to one another, because of its multiplanar imaging capabilities.

Our experience in musculoskeletal disease has shown that MRI delivers an important contribution to pediatric hip problems, joint diseases, diseases of the vertebral column and above all in staging of musculoskeletal tumors.

In the field of pediatric hip disorders, obstructing factors in congenital dislocation of the hip were studied. MRI reveals information about adherence of the limbus to the capsule and differentiation between eversion or inversion of the limbus.
Subsequently flattening of the femoral head, nonconcentric position of the femoral head in the acetabulum and fluid accumulation in the hip joint can be demonstrated. For this reason MRI plays a prominent part in the selection of the appropriate form of therapy in congenital dislocaton of the hip.
In the irritable hip MRI can differentiate transient synovitis from avascular necrosis of the femoral head (Perthes disease) with the related consequence of treatment.

In the acute traumatized knee joint ruptures of the collateral ligaments, cruciate ligaments as well as meniscal tears can be visualized by MRI in a non-invasive way. In the shoulder joint ruptures of the labrum can be distinguished. The clinical application of MRI in the traumatized joint is still in study. In diseases of the vertebral column MRI visualizes the relation of the vertebral bodies and intravertebral discs in relation to the spinal canal. Further more MRI is helpful in the differentiation between vertebral osteoporosis and metastases.

In the treatment planning of bone tumors information on the stage of the disease is of major importance.
Nowadays limb-saving surgical procedures for malignant bone tumors are increasingly applicated instead of ablative surgery.

Since 1983 we use MRI in the pretreatment staging of all our patients with bone tumors to delineate the extension of the tumor in relation to the anatomy.
It became evident that MRI was very helpful for adequate treatment planning.
MRI is the most accurate staging study in determing the extension of the tumor in relation to the muscle compartments, major vessels and joints.
This visualization is not influenced by the anatomic location of the tumor.
Comparison of the available imaging studies and the tumor specimen confirms that MRI is superior to other imaging studies for questions related to intra-osseous extension, extra-osseous tumor extension, involvement of major vessels and nerves especially in tumors of the pelvis and vertebral column.
Due to the superior information on tumor extension MRI has contributed considerably to the increased number of oncological adequate limb-saving procedures.

In patients with malignant bone tumors MRI is indispensable, especially when limbsaving surgery is considered because of its exact delineation on intra- and extra-osseous tumor extension.

Superior soft tissue contrast, flexible image planes and vascular imaging in relation to pathology are responsible for the increased value of MRI in the field of musculoskeletal disease.

REFERENCES

Bloem J.L., Taminiau A.H.M., Kieft G.J., et al: MRI van het Steun- en Bewegingsapparaat. NTVG 1987, in press.

Bloem J.L., Falke T.H.M., Taminiau A.H.M., et al: MRI of Primary Malignant Bone Tumors. Radiographics 1985; 5: 853-886.

Bloem J.L., Bluemm R.G., Taminiau A.H.M. et al: MRI of Primary Malignant Bone Tumors. Radiographics 1987; 7,3:425-445

Bos C.F.A., Bloem J.L., Obermann W.R. et al: Magnetic Resonance Imaging in congenital dislocation of the hip. J Bone Joint Surg, in press.

Index